RARE DISORDERS RESEARCH PROGRESS

Additional books and e-books in this series can be found on Nova's website under the Series tab.

RARE DISORDERS RESEARCH PROGRESS

VESTIBULAR SCHWANNOMA

PATHOPHYSIOLOGY, DIAGNOSIS AND TREATMENT

FRANCESCO DISPENZA, MD, PHD
AND
FRANCESCO MARTINES, MD, PHD
EDITORS

nova
Medicine & Health
New York

Additional color graphics may be available in the e-book version of this book.

Library of Congress Cataloging-in-Publication Data

ISBN: 978-1-53617-191-4
Names: Dispenza, Francesco, editor. | Martines, Francesco (Associate professor), editor.
Title: Vestibular schwannoma : pathophysiology, diagnosis and treatment / [edited by Francesco Dispenza, Francesco Martines].
Identifiers: LCCN 2019059668 (print) | LCCN 2019059669 (ebook) | ISBN 9781536171914 (hardcover) | ISBN 9781536171921 (adobe pdf)
Subjects: LCSH: Acoustic neuroma.
Classification: LCC RC280.E2 V47 2019 (print) | LCC RC280.E2 (ebook) | DDC 616.99/385--dc23
LC record available at https://lccn.loc.gov/2019059668
LC ebook record available at https://lccn.loc.gov/2019059669

Published by Nova Science Publishers, Inc. † New York

CONTENTS

PREFACE

Vestibular schwannoma is a rare benign tumor arising from VIII cranial nerve. Its localisation into internal auditory canal and cerebello-pontine angle is the main reason for the relevant clinical implication of such disease.

This book develops all the features regarding the vestibular schwannoma, starting from the biology of the tumor, passing to the clinical presentation and instrumental diagnostic pathway to make diagnosis and concluding with therapeutic options linked to several factors regarding tumor size, localisation, symptoms, patient characteristics and outcome.

The chapters are divided into 3 sections: pathophysiology, clinical features and treatment.

Advancements in microsurgical technique and radiosurgery, coupled with an increased understanding of the natural history of the disease, have made modern management of this tumor considerably more complex and the opinions are still divided between conservatism and definitive cure.

The last section includes the rehabilitation after treatment of patients affected by vestibular schwannoma.

The contributions to this book were done by several eminent expert authors in their field, and all references are up to date. This is a robust resource for residents, fellows, and early attending physicians, as well as mid- to later-career physicians who care for patients with vestibular schwannoma.

Chapter 1 - Vestibular schwannomas (VS) are benign slow growing tumors, arising from the VIII cranial nerve, generally involving the inferior vestibular nerve. This tumor could be part of a systemic disease called Neurofibromatosis type 2 (NF2), in which the tumors are bilateral and more aggressive. The identification of prognostic factor should help the otoneurologist in selecting a proper management. Whereas radiological features and presenting symptoms did not result good prognostic factor or predictor element of tumor development, molecular elements, as well as microRNA, could be useful to act as predictive factors of biological behavior of VS in time. It is clear that miR-21 plays a significant role in the regulation of multiple pathways controlling cell proliferation in many cancers, and this attribute makes it a very attractive target for the development of new therapies. Future experiments aimed at manipulating miR-21 expression in schwannoma models will allow us to test the relative importance of miR-21 on VS growth in vivo. The close relationship between growth and miR-21 expression lead to considerate such molecular factor as a prognostic indicator, after further verifications, to select patients manageable with observation or with an early hearing preservation surgery.

Chapter 2 - Vestibular schwannoma (VS) is a benign, slow-growing tumor of the vestibulocochlear nerve. It comprises around 80% of cerebellopontine angle tumors. VS usually presents with hearing loss but can also cause vestibular hypofunction, balance disturbances, and vertigo. The ischemia caused by the compromise of the cochlear blood supply and mass effects caused by the growing tumor have been proposed as a mechanism of audio-vestibular dysfunction.

Presenting symptoms can include unilateral hearing loss, tinnitus, vertigo and/or balance disturbances, facial (VII) or trigeminal (V) nerve dysfunction and neurosurgical signs and symptoms. Magnetic resonance imaging (MRI) is considered the gold standard to diagnose VS. The clinical workup normally includes also the pure tone audiometry, speech discrimination testing, auditory brainstem response (ABR) test and, to a lesser extent, a vestibular function testing. Despite the relatively high sensitivity achieved by combining multiple tests, imaging has always been decisive in demonstrating the presence of a space-occupying lesion in the cerebellopontine angle. So, the role of audiovestibular examinations has been restricted, merely providing arguments to proceed to some type of imaging.

Chapter 3 - Neurofibromatosis type 2 (NF2) is a rare neurocutaneous disorder characterised by bilateral vestibular schwannomas associated with meningiomas, ependymomas and other cranial nerve and peripheral schwannomas. The clinical manifestations of NF2 show varying degrees of severity and age-related differences. Childhood presentation of NF2 also predicts a severe disease course. NF2 is genetically caused by germ-line mutations of the *NF2* gene located on 22q12.17. The *NF2* gene encodes a protein called merlin. Merlin associates with several transmembrane receptors and intracellular proteins serving as a tumor-suppressor. The diagnosis of NF2 is established based on clinical criteria, or combined molecular and clinical criteria. Specific genotype and phenotype correlations have been identified so far. Although significant progress in neurosurgery, radio-surgery and auditory rehabilitation have increased the treatment options for individuals with NF2, these show higher mortality rates than in the general population. Thus, tumour surveillance remains the cornerstone of NF2 patient management. Recent advances in the elucidation of the role of merlin have led to the development of biological targeted therapies.

Chapter 4 - Lesions of the cerebellopontine angle and internal auditory canal are a frequent finding in neuroradiological examinations and their detection may represent a diagnostic challenge. Among these lesions, vestibular schwannomas and meningiomas are certainly the most frequent and account for up to 90% of all cerebellopontine angle tumours. The remaining ones are a group of lesions arising from the different structures found in these anatomical regions such as haemangiomas, lipomas, lymphomas, facial nerve tumours, and aneurysms. This chapter will introduce this topic focusing on a practical coverage of the typical and atypical neuroradiological signs that will drive towards the most correct differential diagnosis checklist. High-quality neuroradiological images will support the reader for an optimal learning experience.

Chapter 5 - Therapeutic strategies of vestibular schwannomas treatment are changed in the last years. The improvement of surgical equipments and skills allowed increasing the *number* of successful operations in the last 10 years. The results improved in terms of survival, quality of life, recurrences, facial nerve function, and hearing preservation Also, the age of operated patients, once a restriction, becomes progressively a relative limitation to surgical indication.

However, the progressive widening of MRI availability gives to the Otoneurologist the possibility to follow-up the patients with a *relatively* simple radiological examination, delaying the decision to treat surgically the neoplasm only in case of growth or symptoms occurrence.

The medical society is in demand of a treatment strategy based on hard data especially on the growth pattern of these tumors.

To have a complete picture of the treatment options the authors will discuss following the several *modalities* to manage a solitary vestibular schwannoma; the discussion about radiotherapy-radiosurgery is treated elsewhere in this book.

Chapter 6 - Conservative management means a low-morbidity control of disease with long term preservation of function and no post-treatment sequelae. It relates, daresay only, to small-size vestibular schwannoma. The "small size" tumor is defined as a less or equal to 10mm lesion in the cerebello-pontine angle, the Koos classification being not representative and rarely used in the otological community. The more the size increases, the less the conservative management can be successful. A balance between different conditions at diagnosis and between the pros and contra of each option has to be considered. The conservative treatment of a small tumor relates today to the possibility of hearing preservation, the choice to treat or not treat the tumor cannot leave this out of consideration. The conservative treatment means also low morbidity treatment, and there should be a better definition of what today morbidity for a small tumor is.

Chapter 7 - The translabyrinthine approach (TLA) is a transpetrosal surgical approach to the cerebellopontine angle (CPA). In this approach the mastoid and posterior labyrinth are removed in order to expose the middle and posterior fossa dura and the internal auditory canal (IAC) lying immediately medial to the labyrinth itself. The idea behind the approach is to take advantage of the medial extension of the temporal bone in order to reach the CPA through the shortest route and with no or only minimal cerebellar manipulation. Theoretically the enlarged TLA allows removal of posterior fossa neoplasm of any dimensions; however, some anatomical variations of the temporal bone may require appropriate management.

Chapter 8 - The retrosigmoid approach has been widely described and utilized for access to various pathologies of the posterior fossa and the cerebellopontine angle. This approach gives a better view of the CPA and allows early identification of various neurovascular structures, more complete removal of lesions, less morbidity, and better functional results in terms of cochlear and facial nerve preservation. Many authors advocate it as the procedure of choice during vestibular nerve section, microvascular decompression, surgery for vestibular schwannomas, non-acoustic tumors, or insertion of auditory brain stem implants.

Chapter 9 - The Middle Fossa Approach (MFA) is ideally used for hearing preservation in relatively young patients with small intracanalicular VS with serviceable hearing, especially when there is lateral extension of the VS into the fundus of the IAC. MFA provides a short surgical corridor to approach the tumour with minimal manipulation of the cranial nerves VII and VIII, thus reducing the odds of cranial nerves impairment. Significant tumour extension medially into the cisternal space of the cerebellopontine angle is considered a limitation to this approach.

Chapter 10 - Endoscopic approach is an alternative surgical technique developed for the management of VSs limited to the IAC, minimizing intraoperative and postoperative complications.

After several cadaver dissections to better understand the anatomy and to define appropriate instruments for the surgery, some advances were made in exploring the inner ear: from the labyrinth, jugular, and carotid to the IAC, until an appropriate procedure was recorded and ready to be applied clinically.

Improving the experience in endoscopic ear surgery, the most important advantage in performing surgery in these tumors with endoscopic approach was the reduction of postoperative morbility, that was comparable to that of a tympanoplasty rather than an operation of the CPA. In conclusion, in the author's opinion, the transcanal surgery, with TTEA and/or ETA technique, can be added in the "decision making" algorhytm for the management of VS.

Chapter 11 - The role of radiotherapy for the treatment of VS has been established since the first Gamma-knife radiosurgery experiences took place in 1969. The constant progress of technology allowed the development of more accurate systems able to ensure the safe irradiation of deep located lesions, inaccessible for neurosurgery, with a reduced risk of radiation-related damages. This led to consider the use of radiation therapy an iso-effective alternative to surgery, with a smaller impact on neurological sequelae. Nowadays, radiotherapy for VS can be delivered with stereotactic radiosurgery, conventional fractionation, hypofraction-ation and particle therapy.

Chapter 12 - Facial nerve (FN) palsy represents the most frequent complication of VS surgery, therefore all of the professionals involved in the treatment of VS should be aware of its implications and treatment. Several treatments have been described for the management of facial nerve paralysis. The choice of the repair technique depends on various factors, including the type and site of lesion, the time elapsed from the injurious event, the patient's expectations and the rehabilitation. Post-operative facial nerve paralysis can be treated with static and dynamic techniques.

Static techniques are based on the passive correction of muscle deficits without restoring their movement, while dynamic techniques aim to restore the active function of the affected mimic muscles, through the restoration of the muscular innervation or their replacement with free or pedunculated muscle flaps.

Chapter 13 - Rehabilitation therapy can be used to treat balance disorders via exercises organized into anatomo-pathological protocols. In general, there is an indication for rehabilitation whenever compensation of a patient's vestibular system fails to adequately resolve spontaneously.

Although the therapeutical indications have expanded over time, it is especially useful to treat balance disorders in neurological patients and those with acute damage to the vestibular system. Specifically, it favors and accelerates spontaneous central compensation in a variety of neurological disorders such as Multiple Sclerosis, Parkinson's disease, cerebellar pathologies or in brain tumors like Vestibular Schwannoma (or Acoustic Neurinoma). The latter is a benign intracranial tumor that affects the acoustic nerve (or cranial nerve VIII), which is concerned with hearing, balance and head position. It represents about 6% of all intracranial tumors, with an incidence of approximately 1 per 100,000 person-years. Affected patients present with a range of symptoms including discomfort, reduced motor capacity and afflictions that lead to functional limitations in the activities of daily life and personal care, especially in performing tasks requiring some degree of postural balance. The aim is to treat them through a series of exercises to be repeated both with the aid of a specialized supervisor and unassisted at home; the treatment is based on proprioceptive and vestibular exercises that progressively improve their quality of life.

In: Vestibular Schwannoma
Editors: Francesco Dispenza et al.
ISBN: 978-1-53617-191-4

Chapter 1

BIOLOGY OF VESTIBULAR SCHWANNOMA: THE ROLE OF PTEN AND MICRORNA-21

Francesco Dispenza[1,2], MD, PhD,
Sebastiano Puglisi[2], MD and Angelo Immordino[2], MD
[1]Euro Mediterranean Institute of Science and Technology - IEMEST, Palermo, Italy
[2]U. O. C. Otorhinolaryngology University Hospital Policlinico P. Giaccone, Palermo, Italy

ABSTRACT

Vestibular schwannomas (VS) are benign slow growing tumors, arising from the VIII cranial nerve, generally involving the inferior vestibular nerve. This tumor could be part of a systemic disease called Neurofibromatosis type 2 (NF2), in which the tumors are bilateral and more aggressive. The identification of prognostic factor should help the otoneurologist in selecting a proper management. Whereas radiological features and presenting symptoms did not result good prognostic factor or predictor element of tumor development, molecular elements, as well as microRNA, could be useful to act as predictive factors of biological behavior of VS in time. It is clear that miR-21 plays a significant role in the regulation of multiple pathways controlling cell proliferation in many cancers, and this attribute makes it a very attractive target for the development of new therapies. Future experiments aimed at manipulating miR-21 expression in schwannoma models will allow us to test the relative importance of miR-21 on VS growth in vivo. The close relationship between growth and miR-21 expression lead to considerate such molecular factor as a prognostic indicator, after further verifications, to select patients manageable with observation or with an early hearing preservation surgery.

INTRODUCTION

Vestibular schwannomas (VS) are benign slow growing tumors, arising from the VIII cranial nerve, generally involving the inferior vestibular nerve. This tumor could be part of a systemic disease called Neurofibromatosis type 2 (NF2), in which the tumors are bilateral and more aggressive. Vestibular schwannomas represent about 6% of all intracranial tumors and accounts for about 80% of all tumors diagnosed in the cerebello-pontine angle (CPA). The incidence reported is 10-20:1000000 per year [1]. The incidence apparently increased in the last 10 years, but it was due to the enlarged availability of MRI done for other reasons. However, the true incidence could be different and greater than known, because of a lot of tumors remain silent and undiagnosed. Certainly, the unpredictable behavior of the tumor is a concern in choosing a treatment plan that is generally consequent to: hearing status, tumor size, and performance status of patient. The identification of prognostic factor should help the otoneurologist in selecting a proper management. Whereas radiological features and presenting symptoms did not result good prognostic factor or predictor element of tumor development, molecular elements, as well as microRNA, could be useful to act as predictive factors of biological behavior of VS in time.

MicroRNA-21 and PTEN Pathway

The discovery of microRNAs has broadened our understanding of the mechanism that control gene expression with the addition of an entirely novel level of regulatory control. These small noncoding transcripts of 18-25 nucleotides modulate protein expression by binding to complementary or partially complementary target mRNAs, and thereby targeting the mRNA for degradation or translational inhibition [2]. Mature microRNA binds to specific mRNA targets in region complementary to the microRNA and, by a mechanism that is not completely understood, resulting in translational repression or degradation of the mRNA9.

It has been demonstrated that tumors exhibit aberrant microRNA expression profiles, indicating that such molecules play an important role in cellular differentiation, development, metabolism, apoptosis, and cancer [3].

MicroRNA-21 (miR-21) has been founded overexpressed in many tumors including: breast, liver, and glioblastoma [4, 5]. One of the targets of miR-21 was identified as mRNA encoding for phosphatase and tensin homolog (PTEN), a tumor suppressor [5].

PTEN is the most highly mutated tumor-suppressor gene in the post-p53 era; it plays a role not only in inducing cell cycle arrest and programming apoptosis, but also in other aspects of cell physiology, including cell adhesion, migration and differentiation. Decreased expression of PTEN would enhance proliferative signaling through the pathway of AKT regulation, by activating this kinase, and finally leading to proliferation, decreased apoptosis or both. The PI3K/AKT signaling pathway is a growth-promoting system in several human malignant tumors. AKT has been involved in cell survival and growth, in differentiation and apoptosis as well [6]. PI3K is a membrane-associated lipid kinase that catalyzes the conversion of phosphatidylinositol diphosphate (PIP2) to phosphatidylinositol triphosphate (PIP3). This event recruits AKT from the cytoplasm to the membrane to a direct action between PIP3 and AKT [6]. The activation of AKT is mediated by phosphoinositide-dependent protein kinase (PDK) by phosphorylation of an AKT site; a second phosphorylation is required for a maximal activation [7]. The principal negative regulator of AKT activation is PTEN, which role consists in the conversion of PIP3 in PIP2. PIP3 levels are very low in quiescent cells, but rapidly increase upon stimulation by growth factors, through activation of PI3K, as mentioned.

Generally, a loss of the PTEN function is secondary to a deletion on chromosome 10, but in low grade glioneural tumors PTEN mutation are rare, hence is the regulation of its activity that is deregulated. PTEN have opposite function of PI3K in regulating cell proliferation and survival by regulation of PDK phosphorylation state. The activity of PTEN is also regulated by a phosphorylation that decreases its phosphatase activity.

The Role of MicroRNA-21 and PTEN in Cancer Development

The study of miRNA in VS originates by the observation of its behavior and effects in other tumors. Perturbations in AKT signaling have been shown to induce malignant transformation in ovarian cancer, lymphomas, pancreatic cancer, hepatocellular carcinoma, gastric cancer, prostatic cancer, and thyroid cancer [8].

Inhibition of miR-21 in hepatocellular carcinoma cell lines increased expression of tumor suppressor PTEN and decreased cellular proliferation, migration and invasion, whereas enhancing miR-21 expression caused opposite effects [5]. In breast cancer was showed that transfection of cells lines with anti-miR-21 resulted in increased apoptosis and inhibition of cell growth [9]. Also in VS cell cultures the proliferative rate and the cell survival was downregulated by a same procedure, indicating that miR-21 have a similar role [10]. In colorectal cancer has been demonstrated that the tumor suppressor PDCD4 (programmed cell death 4) is a target of miR-21 and its downregulation stimulated invasion, extravasation and metastasis [11].

In primary brain tumors high levels of miR-21 were founded, with maximum overexpression in glioblastomas [4]. MicroRNA-21 might block the expression of gene products that promote normal glia differentiation or that induce apoptosis, holding tumor cells in an inappropriately primitive and proliferative developmental state. Schwann cells are part of the glia tissue, hence may exhibit some deregulation of miR-21 expression in tumor cases as well. MicroRNA-21 overexpression in VS may become, consequently, a key point in the control of growth and development by PTEN regulation and its effects, as stated before, on AKT pathway.

MicroRNA-21, PTEN and Vestibular Schwannoma

The importance of miR-21 role in VS growth is showed by a linear correlation between expression and size at time of diagnosis. Furthermore, an interesting relationship emerged between miR-21 expression and growth rate that seems to be related with the level of miR-21, opening the perspective to perform an early hearing preservation surgery in those patients with high risk of tumor growth.

The protein PTEN acts as tumor suppressor inhibiting phosphoinositide 3-kinase/protein kinase B (PI3K/AKT) pathway that promotes cell proliferation, cell survival and tumor growth [12]. The PI3K/AKT pathway was founded activated in human VS development. The activation of antiapoptotic growth-promoting pathways such as the PI3K/AKT system may be a key mechanism whereby tumors gain a survival advantage [13]. Increased levels of miR-21 in VS have a determinant role in downregulating PTEN expression and, as consequence, hyperactivating AKT signal, input to VS development.

The deregulation of proliferation activity and cell apoptosis lead to tumor formation and growth is often associated with mutation of the NF2 gene, which encodes the tumor suppressor protein called "merlin." This mutation is constitutionally present in NF2 patients, while is often acquired in sporadic VS. Whereas the merlin alteration is well known in NF2, the development mechanism of the solitary VS was only recently studied.

Merlin, the protein product for the NF2 gene, is structurally similar to the ezrin/radixin/moesin cytoskeletal proteins, but has unique tumor-suppressive properties [14]. Overexpression of merlin suppresses growth of rat schwannoma cells, whereas merlin inactivation leads to loss of contact inhibition and increased cell proliferation [15]. The merlin regulate also the PI3K activation through its interaction with an enhancer, consequently and indirectly acts as a suppressor of the AKT pathway activation [16]. The merlin was founded mutated in sporadic VS with loss its biological function in 53-70% of examined cases [17].

As showed by Scoles et al., merlin protein play a role in suppressing STAT3 (signal transducer and activator of transcription 3) activation through interaction with hepatocyte growth factor-regulated tyrosine kinase substrate (HRS) in human schwannoma cell line [18]. STAT3, which is a regulator of gene expression in response to many growth factors and cytokines, induces expression of miR-21 [19]. In fact, the microRNA-21 gene presents an upstream enhancer region containing two binding sites for STAT3. The mutation occurring in NF2 patients interferes with binding of HRS with merlin abolishing the ability of merlin to inhibit STAT3 activation. This open the possibility that overexpression of miR-21 in VS may be a consequence of a deregulated activation of STAT3 by an autocrine or paracrine mechanism involving neuropoietic cytokines [10].

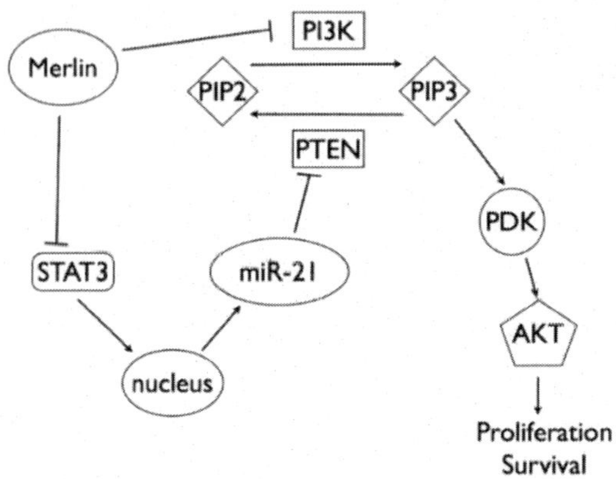

Figure 1. Schematic pathway showing the role of the main factors that induce cell proliferation and/or survival. Overexpression of mRNA-21 cause inhibition of PTEN that have the main role in down regulation of the AKT.

STAT3 is activated also by the neuropoietic cytokines IL-6 playing an important role in nerve repair and regeneration [20]. The activation of STAT signaling is regulated even by epidermal growth factor receptor (EGFR) pathway, which contribute to cell proliferation in tumoral cell of NF2 patients and in primary VS cultures [21]. This mechanism is not clear, but the use of a EGFR inhibitor in NF2 subjects showed some benefit in term of arrest of growth [22], although not statistically proved, the targeted therapy hold some promise. Probably other mRNA that may be targeted by miR-21 may either serve unrelated functions or may serve to modulate the effect of PTEN. Based on target prediction algorithms, PTEN potentially could be targeted by miRNA other than miR-21, but PTEN needs to be verified experimentally as a good target for these miRNAs, and a biologically relevant role shown.

The cystic phenotype of VS was indicated as more aggressive form of tumor, because of the accumulation of fluid into cyst may determine a rapid expansion of the mass, compressing rapidly the surrounding structures [23]. MicroRNA-21 increases matrix metalloproteinase-2 (MM2) expression in cardiac fibroblasts by the PTEN pathway, and MM2 has been associated with cyst formation in VS [24]. It has been shown that the cystic type of VS exhibits a higher expression of miR-21 compared with solid type and it is presumable that the cyst formation has a close relationship with the overexpression of miR-21.

Recently, it was discovered that extracellular miRNAs circulate in the blood of both healthy and diseased patients, although ribonuclease is present in both plasma and serum [25]. Most of the circulating miRNAs are included in lipid or lipoprotein complexes, such as apoptotic bodies, microvesicles, or exosomes, and are, therefore, highly stable. The existence of circulating miRNAs in the blood of cancer patients has raised the possibility that miRNAs may serve as a novel diagnostic marker. However, the secretory mechanism and biological function, as well as the meaning of the existence of extracellular miRNAs, remain largely unclear. These findings may resolve the problem of difficulty access to VS specimen to analyze preoperatively the miR-21 levels and, consequently, establish a prognosis.

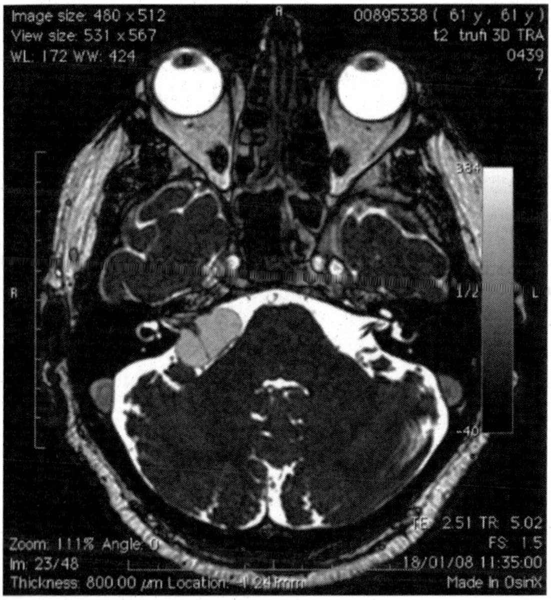

Figure 2. MRI axial scan T2-weighted showing a cystic vestibular schwannoma. The cystic component is the prevalent portion displayed with an intermediate gray due to difference in proteins content compared to cerebrospinal fluid.

CONCLUSION

It is clear that miR-21 plays a significant role in the regulation of multiple pathways controlling cell proliferation in many cancers, and this attribute makes it a very attractive target for the development of new therapies. Future experiments aimed at manipulating miR-21 expression in schwannoma models will allow us to test the relative importance of miR-21 on VS growth in vivo. The close relationship between growth and miR-21 expression lead to considerate such molecular factor as a prognostic indicator, after further verifications, to select patients manageable with observation or with an early hearing preservation surgery.

Furthermore, the application of proteomics strategies in these cells should help identify new molecular targets of miR-21 as has been demonstrated in the breast cancer cell line [26, 27]. The application of these methods and findings in other biologic systems may shed new light on the molecular pathways controlling tumor growth and help identify novel therapeutic targets for the treatment of VS.

Should miR-21 be confirmed to be integral to the growth and regulation of VS, it is possible to clinically manipulate this biologic phenomenon. Using molecules that can bind and interfere with these microRNAs, would be one strategy to downregulate this pathway. Early clinical trials using this approach have been used in patients with macular degeneration and respiratory syncytial virus infections [28-33]. A miR-21 specific RNA interference knockdown could be achieved systemically by administering a viral gene expression vector; however, the side effects on a patient may be undesirable because of off target effects. A more focused delivery via an endoscopic direct injection or delivery during an intentionally incomplete resection of the VS could be an alternative method.

REFERENCES

[1] Stangerup, S. E., Caye-Thomasen, P., Tos, M., Thomsen, J. The Natural History of Vestibular Schwannoma. *Otol. Neurotol.* 2006;27:547-552.

[2] Bartel, D. P. MicroRNAs: genomics, biogenesis, mechanism, and function. *Cell* 2004;116:281-297.

[3] Hwang, H. W., Mendell, J. T. MicroRNAs in cell proliferation, cell death, and tumorigenesis. *Br. J. Cancer* 2006;94:776-780.

[4] Chan, J. A., Krichevsky, A. M., Kosik, K. S. MicroRNA-21 is an antiapoptotic factor in human glioblastoma cells. *Cancer Res.* 2005;65:6029-6033.

[5] Meng, F., Henson, R., Wehbe-Janek, H., Ghoshal, K., Jacob, S. T., Patel, T. MicroRNA-21 regulates expression of the PTEN tumor suppressor gene in human hepatocellular cancer. *Gastroenterology* 2007;133:647-658.

[6] Toker, A., Newton, A. C. Cellular signaling: pivoting around PDK-1. *Cell* 2000;103:185-188.

[7] Mora, A., Komander, D., van Aalten, D. M., et al. PDK1, the master regulator of AGC kinase signal transduction. *Semin. Cell Dev. Biol.* 2004;15:161-170.

[8] Altomare, D. A., Testa, J. R. Perturbations of the AKT signaling pathway in human cancer. *Oncogene* 2005;24:7455-7464.

[9] Si, M. L., Zhu, S., Wu, H., Lu, Z., Wu, F., Mo, Y. Y. miR-21-mediated tumor growth. *Oncogene* 2007;26:2799-2803.

[10] Cioffi, J. A., Yue, W. Y., Mendolia-Loffredo, S., Hansen, K. R., Wackym, P. A., Hansen, M. R. MicroRNA-21 overexpression contributes to vestibular schwannoma cell proliferation and survival. *Otol. Neurotol.* 2010.

[11] Asangani, I. A., Rasheed, S. A., Nikolova, D. A., et al. MicroRNA-21 (miR-21) post-transcriptionally downregulates tumor suppressor Pdcd4 and stimulates invasion, intravasation and metastasis in colorectal cancer.

[12] Di Cristofano, A., Pandolfi, P. P. The multiple roles of PTEN in tumor suppression. *Cell* 2000;100:387-390.

[13] Jacob, A., Lee, T. X., Neff, B. A., Miller, S., Welling, B., Chang, L. S. Phosphatidylinositol 3-kinase/AKT pathway activation in human vestibular schwannoma. *Otol. Neurotol.* 2008;29:58-68.

[14] Trofatter, J. A., MacCollin, M. M., Rutter, J. L., et al. A novel moesin-, ezrin-, radixin-like gene is a candidate for the neurofibromatosis 2 tumor suppressor. *Cell* 1993;72:791-800.

[15] Huynh, D. P., Pulst, S. M. Neurofibromatosis 2 antisense oligodeoxynucleotides induce reversible inhibition of schwannomin synthesis and cell adhesion in STS26T and T98G cells. *Oncogene* 1996;13:73-84.

[16] Rong, R., Xiaoling, T., Gutmann, D. H., et al. Neurofibromatosis 2 (NF2) tumor suppressor merlin inhibits phosphatidylinositol 3-kinase through binding to PIKE-L. *PNAS* 2004;101:18200-18205.

[17] Neff, B. A., Welling, D. B., Akhmametyeva, E. M., Chang, L. S. The molecular biology of vestibular schwannomas: dissecting the

pathogenic process at the molecular level. *Otol. Neurotol.* 2006;27:197-208.

[18] Scoles, D. R., Nguyen, V. D., Qin, Y., et al. Neurofibromatosis 2 (NF2) tumor suppressor schwannomin and its interacting protein HRS regulate STAT signaling. *Hum. Mol. Genet.* 2002;11:3179-3189.

[19] Loffler, D., Brocke-Heidrich, K., Pfeifer, G., et al. Interleukin-6 dependent survival of multiple myeloma cells involves the Stat3-mediated induction of microRNA-21 through a highly conserved enhancer. *Blood* 2007;110:1330-1333.

[20] Ernst, M., Jenkins, B. J. Acquiring signalling specificity from the cytokine receptor gp130. *Trends Genet.* 2004;20:23-32.

[21] Hansen, M. R., Roehm, P. C., Chatterjee, P., Green, S. H. Constitutive neuregulin-1/ErbB signaling contributes to human vestibular schwannoma proliferation. *Glia* 2006;53:593-600.

[22] Plotkin, S. R., Halpin, C., McKenna, M. J., Loeffler, J. S., Batchelor, T. T., Barker, F. G., 2nd. Erlotinib for progressive vestibular schwannoma in neurofibromatosis 2 patients. *Otol. Neurotol.* 2010;31:1135-1143.

[23] Piccirillo, E., Wiet, M. R., Flanagan, S., et al. Cystic Vestibular Schwannoma: Classification, Management and Facial Nerve Outcomes. *Otol. Neurotol.* 2009;30:826-834.

[24] Moon, K. S., Jung, S., Seo, S. K. et al. Cystic vestibular schwannomas: a possible role of matrix metalloproteinase-2 in cyst development and unfavorable surgical outcome. *J. Neurosurg.* 2007;106:866-871.

[25] Kosaka, N., Iguchi, H., Ochiya, T. Circulating microRNA in body fluid: a new potential biomarker for cancer diagnosis and prognosis. *Cancer Science*; 101:2087-2092.

[26] Livak, K. J., Schmittgen, T. D. Analysis of relative gene expression data using real-time quantitative PCR and the 2(jDelta Delta C(T)) method. *Methods* 2001;25:402-408.

[27] Yang, Y., Chaerkady, R., Beer, M. A., et al. Identification of miR-21 targets in breast cancer cells using a quantitative proteomic approach. *Proteomics* 2009;9:1374-1384.

[28] Sah, D. W. Therapeutic potential of RNA interference for neurological disorders. *Life Sci*. 2006;79:1773-1780.

[29] Di Stadio, A., Dipietro, L., Toffano, R., Burgio, F., De Lucia, A., Ippolito, V., Garofalo, S., Ricci, G., Martines, F., Trabalzini, F., Della Volpe, A. (2018) Working memory function in children with single side deafness using a bone-anchored hearing implant: A case-control study. *Audiology and Neurotology*, 23 (4), pp. 238-244.

[30] Scorpecci, A., Massoud, M., Giannantonio, S., Zangari, P., Lucidi, D., Martines, F., Foligno, S., Di Felice, G., Minozzi, A., Luciani, M., Marsella, P. (2018) Otogenic lateral sinus thrombosis in children: proposal of an experience-based treatment flowchart. *European Archives of Oto-Rhino-Laryngology,* 275 (8), pp. 1971-1977.

[31] Dispenza, F., Battaglia, A. M., Salvago, P., Martines, F. Determinants of failure in the reconstruction of the tympanic membrane: a case-control study. *Iranian Journal Otorhinolaryngology*, 2018; 30:341-346.

[32] Dispenza, F., De Stefano, A., Costantino, C., Rando, D., Giglione, M., Stagno, R., Bennici, E. Canal switch and re-entry phenomenon in benign paroxysmal positional vertigo: difference between immediate and delayed occurrence. *Acta Otorhinolaryngol. Ital.* 2015; 35:116-120.

[33] Dispenza, F., Cappello, F., Kulamarva, G., De Stefano, A. The discovery of the stapes. *Acta Otorhinolaryngol. Ital.* 2015; 33:357-359.

In: Vestibular Schwannoma
Editors: Francesco Dispenza et al.
ISBN: 978-1-53617-191-4

Chapter 2

CLINICAL FEATURES, INSTRUMENTAL AND IMAGING FOR DIAGNOSIS OF VESTIBULAR SCHWANNOMA

Ignazio La Mantia, MD, PhD, Claudio Andaloro, MD and Veronica Castro, MD

Otolayngology Unit, Department of Medical Sciences, Surgical and Advanced Technologies, GF Ingrassia, University of Catania, Catania, Italy

ABSTRACT

Vestibular schwannoma (VS) is a benign, slow-growing tumor of the vestibulocochlear nerve. It comprises around 80% of cerebellopontine angle tumors. VS usually presents with hearing loss but can also cause vestibular hypofunction, balance disturbances, and vertigo. The ischemia caused by the compromise of the cochlear blood supply and mass effects caused by the growing tumor have been proposed as a mechanism of audio-vestibular dysfunction.

Presenting symptoms can include unilateral hearing loss, tinnitus, vertigo and/or balance disturbances, facial (VII) or trigeminal (V) nerve dysfunction and neurosurgical signs and symptoms. Magnetic resonance imaging (MRI) is considered the gold standard to diagnose VS. The clinical workup normally includes also the pure tone audiometry, speech discrimination testing, auditory brainstem response (ABR) test and, to a lesser extent, a vestibular function testing. Despite the relatively high sensitivity achieved by combining multiple tests, imaging has always been decisive in demonstrating the presence of a space-occupying lesion in the cerebellopontine angle. So, the role of audiovestibular examinations has been restricted, merely providing arguments to proceed to some type of imaging.

Keywords: vestibular schwannoma, cerebellopontine angle, unilateral hearing loss, tinnitus, auditory brainstem response, magnetic resonance imaging

Introduction

Vestibular schwannoma (VS) accounts for approximately 80% of cerebellopontine angle tumors. Although it has previously been called acoustic neurinoma, this a misnomer for two reasons. Firstly, the tumor arises from the vestibular division of the vestibulocochlear nerve (VIII cranial nerve), rather than the cochlear division. Secondly, it is derived from the myelin-forming Schwann cells of the associated nerve, rather than the actual neurons (neurinoma). (West et al. 2018, Roosli et al. 2012).

The signs and symptoms of VS are attributed to the involvement of the vestibulocochlear nerve, compressing surrounding cranial nerves, cerebellum, brainstem, as well as raised intracranial pressure. Symptoms are closely correlated with tumor size and often appear as a combination of unilateral sensorineural hearing loss, tinnitus, vertigo and/or disequilibrium. The majority of patients with VS today present with unilateral hearing loss due to cochlear nerve interruption or impairment of blood supply to the nerve. Other clinical features include decreased word understanding, headaches, and facial numbness. In rare cases, with enough growth, VS reaches proportions that cause it to put pressure onto the brainstem, thus affecting other cranial nerves – in particular, the trigeminal nerve – or even vital functions. However, large tumors can still be present but show surprisingly few symptoms and almost no signs except for hearing loss. Even 4-cm and 5-cm tumors may show little physical evidence and display a few of the associated symptoms. (Harner and Laws 1983, Foley et al. 2017).

The diagnosis of vestibular schwannoma (VS) is often made incidentally, during the investigation of other complaints, or as a consequence of patients presenting with otological or neurological symptoms related to VS. Historically, and before the 1980s, the investigation of suspected vestibular schwannomas was focussed upon audio-vestibular investigations supported by plain radiology enhanced with contrast dyes injected into the cerebrospinal fluid. Nowadays, Magnetic resonance imaging (MRI) is considered the gold standard to diagnose VS and is performed whenever there is a high suspicion of VS in patients with the aforementioned symptoms. (Fortnum et al. 2009).

It is, however, a challenge to establish which patients should undergo MRI and which patients should not. Fortunately, there are several tests available that can help to determine whether a patient should be referred for MRI. Pure tone audiometry is usually the first step in the diagnostic process and is sometimes followed by other audiovestibular function tests, such as otoacoustic emissions (OAEs), auditory brainstem response (ABR), caloric irrigation, head impulse test (HIT), and vestibular evoked myogenic potentials (cVEMPs and oVEMPs), All of these tests are important for initial diagnosis as well as subsequent monitoring of disease progression. (Hentschel et al. 2017, von Kirschbaum and Gürkov 2016).

Vestibular Schwannoma Clinical Features

The vestibular nerve, branch of the VIII cranial nerve and origin of the SV, arises from the Pontobulbar junction of the cerebral trunk, crosses the APC and is entered in the CAI accompanied by the VII cranial nerve. The clinic produced by SV is represented by a set of specific symptoms due to its location in the CAI and its growth in the APC.

In the initial stages, in which the SV is confined to the CAI, the symptoms are caused by the direct compression or involvement of the cranial nerves VIII and VII contained in it. As the VSs grow expanding into the tank of the APC, there may be symptoms of compression of the brainstem and V cranial nerve, and if this growth persists it could trigger hydrocephalus and death.

For all these reasons, the evolution of SV has been classified into four different stages depending on the size and location of the tumor. (Selesnick, Jackler and Pitts 1993).

1) Intracanalicular phase: The symptomatology is purely otological (hearing loss, tinnitus, and vertigo).
2) Cisternal phase: The SV can grow without provoking significative alterations in the adjacent structures. It may worsen the otological manifestations and initiate headaches.
3) Compression phase of the brainstem: worsening of the otological manifestations and appearance of signs/symptoms of the V cranial nerve involvement.
4) Hydrocephalus phase: Tumor growth obstructs the IV ventricle causing intracranial hypertension. Headaches, facial weakness, and spasms, loss of visual acuity or diplopia, a wide variety of neural dysfunctions are the main symptoms in this phase till to pyramidal signs and death caused by the cerebral tonsillar herniation.

The reporting of symptoms in the literature at the beginning of 1900 were mainly concerning symptoms of severe neurological involvement and intracranial compression such as papilledema, hydrocephalus, headache, and cerebral dysfunction.

The improvement over time in knowledge of the evolution and symptomatology, diagnostic technologies and treatment capacity allowed diagnosed SVs in more early stages, therefore, paying attention to different signs and symptoms.

Hearing Loss

The hearing loss is the most common symptom of SV and it is characterized by unilateral and progressive hearing loss of sensorineural type.

The literature reports a presence of hearing loss between 85% and 95% in patients with SV. (Kentala and Pyykko 2001).

Generally, hearing loss begins with the deterioration in the acute frequencies and progresses to reach cofosis in some cases, this is thought to occur due to a combination of compression of the cochlear nerve by the growing tumor and a degree of ischemia caused by compromise of the cochlear blood supply (Gouveris, Victor and Mann 2007). On a small proportion of cases (about 2%), hearing loss may be sudden in onset. (Sauvaget et al. 2005).

In common with other sensorineural hearing losses and contrast to conductive hearing loss, the functional hearing loss as measured by speech discrimination thresholds is often more severe than that suggested by pure tone audiometry (Van Dijk, Duijndam and Graamans 2000).

Other hearing patterns may also be present, such as an atypical hearing loss (sudden or fluctuating, which may be mistaken for Meniere's syndrome) or even patient with perfectly normal hearing.

Tinnitus

Tinnitus is the second most commonly reported symptom and will usually occur in combination with hearing loss. The tinnitus typically presented by patients with SV is unilateral with acute and continuous tones, although these characteristics may vary. It has an incidence that oscillates, according to statistics, from 60 to 80% of cases. There is also the case of a small proportion of patients who reported unilateral tinnitus in the absence of subjective hearing loss. (Bakkouri et al. 2009).

The mechanism that provokes it is believed to be the same that causes hearing loss, neural or vascular compression. However, since it is the initial symptom in 10-15% of cases, it is always opportune to exclude a retrocochlear pathology.

Balance Dysfunction/Vertigo

Although the tumor derives from the vestibular nerve, patients infrequently complain of balance disturbances as their primary symptom. Indeed, the incidence of vertigo varies between 18 and 58%. (Stucken, Brown and Selesnick 2012). It is generally accepted that this is because of the slow rate of tumor growth allowing the vestibular system to compensate for a gradual loss of function (Driscoll, 2000).

Vertigo episodes may occur during periods of rapid tumor growth or vascular disorders that alter endogenous compensation mechanisms. Driscoll observes that the symptoms in these patients are probably due to incomplete vestibular compensation, and are rarely significant enough to prompt the patient to seek medical attention. A distinction should be drawn between those patients that present with a small tumor in the internal auditory canal which may cause mild symptoms of imbalance or occasional brief attack of vertigo, and those that present with ataxia due to a large tumor pressing upon the flocculus of the cerebellum: in the latter case, imbalance will often form part of a constellation of neurosurgical symptoms.

Other Cranial Nerves Dysfunction

Other cranial nerves, in particular, the VII (facial) and V (trigeminal) are occasionally affected, with the latter more commonly impaired. The dysfunction of the VII can manifest itself as a hyperfunction (facial spasm) or as a hypofunction (paresis or facial paralysis), they can be present simultaneously. Despite its location, and in contrast to the cochlear nerve, the facial nerve appears to particularly resistant to damage: The House Ear Clinic reported a rate of 2% facial nerve impairment. (Angeli and Jackson 1997).

Another form of involvement of the VII is that of one of its branches, the intermediary nerve of Wrisberg, with alteration of taste in the anterior two-thirds of the tongue, the decrease of the lacrimal secretion and hypesthesia in the area of Ramsay Hunt (sign of Hitselberger). The presence of facial involvement in a small tumor will make it necessary to rule out a primary lesion in the facial nerve.

Trigeminal symptoms are more common, and usually a sign of a larger tumor with a significant cerebellopontine angle component involving the under-surface of the trigeminal nerve as it emerges from the pons. Generally, the sensory roots of the nerve are affected by motor branches intact. Trigeminal nerve dysfunction may be manifested with hyperesthesia, paresthesia, or pain (trigeminal neuralgia) in the malar ipsilateral region to the tumor. Most of the time the patient does not refer to the clinician, but an absent or decreased corneal reflex may be seen at the ocular examination. This involvement of the trigeminal function is related to the tumor size because it is caused by the growth of the SV in the APC. A rate of 16.5% in a surgical series (Mathies and Samii 1997) compares with a rate of 1% in a conservatively managed series (Bakkouri et al. 2009), and this is probably reflecting the larger tumors found among patients undergoing surgery.

Dysfunction or involvement of IX, X, XI, and XII cranial nerves manifests with swallowing disorders, dysphagia, decreased gag reflex, aspiration, dysphonia, and dysarthria. These dysfunctions are caused by the compression of these cranial nerves during the growth of the SV in the APC in the lower and medial direction. They are rare symptoms, as they occur in very advanced stages. The involvement of XII is very rare.

Neurosurgical Symptomatology

In some cases, presentation of the vestibular schwannoma is an emergency, usually due to the development of hydrocephalus. Before the widespread availability of cross-sectional imaging, a significant proportion of patients presented with neurosurgical symptoms; Driscoll reported a headache as a symptom in all 4 patients. (Driscoll 2000). By the latter half of the twentieth century, when cross-sectional imaging was available but limited and the investigation was predominantly audiological, this had reduced to 29% (Mathew et al. 1978) and 38% (Harner and Laws 1981).

It is traditionally accepted that the hydrocephalus seen in vestibular schwannomas is of an obstructive type caused by compression of the 4th ventricle by large tumors. (Driscoll 2000).

Rogg et al. (Rogg et al. 2005) in their paper report a high rate of communicating hydrocephalus (61%), without a strong correlation with tumor volume (as is seen in noncommunicating hydrocephalus). The authors postulate that this sub-clinical hydrocephalus may be related to tumor protein sloughing, but further research is necessary to clarify this.

VESTIBULAR SCHWANNOMA: INSTRUMENTAL AND IMAGING DIAGNOSIS

The annual incidence of diagnosed VS lies around 1/100.000 and is increasing due to an aging population, and the increasing use and sensitivity of magnetic resonance imaging (MRI), which represented the gold standard to diagnose these neoplasms. (Stangerup et al. 2006, De Stefano et al. 2012).

Before MRI was available, VS were diagnosed by performing x-rays, later combined with pneumoventriculography. (Dandy 1918).

Nowadays, MRI is performed whenever there is a high suspicion of VS in patients with the aforementioned symptoms, however, it is a challenge to determine which patients should undergo MRI. In this picture, there are several tests available that can help to determine whether a patient should be referred for MRI. Pure tone audiometry is usually the first step in the diagnostic process and is sometimes followed by other audiovestibular function tests, such as the speech discrimination test, auditory brainstem response, and electronystagmography. (Hentschel et al. 2017).

Audiological Diagnostics

Audiologic examinations are usually the starting point in the diagnostic process.

First, pure tone audiometry (PTA) is applied. PTA scoring indicates the quietest sound detectable by the individual 50% of the time the stimulus is presented. It is performed using an audiometer, and both bone and air conduction are tested at frequencies ranging from 250 to 8000 Hz and at varying intensities ranging from 10–120 decibels hearing level (dbHL). (Paul and Roland 2015).

Results are then represented graphically plotted on an audiogram. Hearing loss is categorized based on the following threshold ranges: mild 26–40dB, moderate 41-55dB, moderately severe 56– 70dB, severe 71–90dB, and profound >90dB. (Clark 1981).

The bone conduction test stimulates the cochlea directly through the mastoid bone and thus, measures noise conduction from the inner ear to the brain. The air conduction test examines the patient's ability to recognize pure tones through the air from the external auditory canal to the brain. The difference between these two measurements is known as the air-bone gap. An audiogram of an individual with sensorineural hearing loss will not show this air-bone gap, rather these patients' audiograms show the same thresholds for air conduction and bone conduction bilaterally. (Paul and Roland 2015).

As previously mentioned, unilateral sensorineural hearing loss is the most common presenting symptom in patients with diagnosed VS. However, there is little agreement in the literature regarding what threshold of asymmetry constitutes the diagnosis. (Margolis and Saly 2008).

Saliba et al. (Saliba et al. 2011) report variability in the reported definition of unilateral sensorineural hearing loss, which can be seen in Table 1.

If on one hand, PTA allows the clinician to determine the type of hearing loss and the level of the hearing impairment on the other its discriminating power is rather poor since it is only able to demonstrate unilateral or asymmetric sensorineural hearing loss, the prominent feature of a VS.

Table 1. Variability on the definition of unilateral sensorineural hearing loss in the literature

Asymmetries	Source
≥ 15 dB at 3,000 Hz	Saliba
≥ 20 dB at any single frequency between 0.5 and 4 kHz	Department of Health
≥ 20 dB at two neighboring frequencies	Sunderland
≥ 15 dB between the average of 0.5, 1, 2 and 3 kHz	AAO-HNS
≥ 15 dB between the average of 0.5 and 8 kHz	Oxford
≥ 15 dB between the average of 1 and 8 kHz	Seattle
≥ 15 dB at any single frequency between 0.5 and 4 kHz	Nashville
≥ 10 dB at two or more frequencies; OR ≥ 15 dB at any single frequency	AMCLASS
≥ 15 dB at two or more frequencies; OR ≥ 15% difference between speech discrimination	Cueva

dB: decibel; kHz: kilohertz.

In addition to the PTA assessment, speech audiometry is also a component of the formal audiologic assessment (Dispenza et al. 2018, Dispenza et al. 2015).

This examination evaluates speech reception, recognition, and understanding. The speech reception threshold (SRT) measures the threshold (in dB) level at which a patient can correctly repeat 50% of spondee words. The number of words that the patient can correctly repeat is presented as a percentage. (Katz et al. 2015).

Gardner-Robertson scoring is used to combine SRT results with patient's corresponding PTA values at frequencies of 500, 1000, and 2000Hz (Table 2), allowing for an objective evaluation of the degree of function hearing impairment suffered by the patient. Test results are graded I to V scale, based on speech discrimination percentage and PTA results. A grade of V indicates deafness, while a grade of I indicates good hearing. (Gardner and Robertson 1988).

Table 2. Gardner-Robertson scoring allows for objective evaluation of the degree of function hearing impairment suffered by the patient

Grade	PTA (dB)	SD (%)
I: Good	0-30	70-100
II: Serviceable	31-50	50-69
III: Non-Serviceable	51-90	5-49
IV: Poor	90-100	1-4
V: Deaf	0	0

db: decibel; PTA: pure tone average; SD: speech discrimination score.

With the Consensus Meeting On Systems For Reporting Results In Vestibular Schwannoma has been introduced a different classification system. The auditory evaluation is done at average frequencies of 500, 1000, and 3000Hz. Speech audiometry was implemented through a score obtained at 40 dB above the threshold of first auditory sensation (FAS). Class A corresponds to a tonal threshold between 0 and 20 dB and a FAS between 80 and 100%; class B has a lower limit of 30 dB of tonal threshold and 70% of FAS. Class C has a lower limit of 40 dB of tonal threshold and 60% of FAS. Class D has a limit of 60 dB and 50%, finally, class E 80 dB and 40%. (Kanzaki et al. 2003).

The speech recognition score (SRS) or word recognition score (WRS) presents patients with 50 monosyllabic words at an intensity level within their detectable range of hearing relative to the SRT or PTA thresholds. The WRS of an individual with normal hearing is expected to be >90% when the individual is presented with words 30dB higher than their SRT. The SRS is often judged excellent to good in patients with conductive hearing loss when the presentation intensity is adequate to reach the cochlea. However, patients with sensorineural hearing loss will generally show reduced performance when the threshold level is increased beyond that which is needed for maximum WRS. This is known as the "rollover" effect, and it is especially evident when testing individuals with sensorineural hearing loss of retrocochlear etiology versus an individual with sensorineural hearing loss of cochlear etiology. (Katz et al. 2015).

Acoustic Brainstem Response

Acoustic brainstem response (ABR) can be used as a further screening test, and before MRI imaging was the most accurate screening tool for suspected VS. This non-invasive test uses scalp electrodes and a click-stimulus administered in the external auditory canal to track the evoked electrical potentials along the auditory nerve fibers from CN VIII as they leave the cochlea and travel to the brain. (Stucken, Brown and Selesnick 2012).

The recorded pathway is visualized as five waveforms, each with anatomical correlates. An interruption of the evoked signal at any point along the pathway would result in latency in the most prominent wave V when compared with the contralateral waveform. Typically, a vestibular schwannoma demonstrates:

- The absence of any reproducible wave, even keeping the hearing threshold
- The presence of an isolated I wave from the unsynchronized traced reminder.
- An extension of the I-III interval greater than 2.5 ms
- An extension of the I-V interval greater than 4.4 ms
- An interaural latency difference of the V wave greater than 0.25 ms
- An interaural difference of the I-V interval greater than 0.2 ms. (Paulraj et al. 2015, Hentschel et al. 2017).

The sensitivity of ABR was reported initially to be more than 90% for the detection of VS, Subsequent studies assessing the sensitivity of auditory brainstem response measurement concludes that, while sensitive for large tumors, the technique is less successful for smaller tumors. (Fortnum et al. 2009).

Pooled results produce sensitivity values of 79%, 95% and 98% for tumours sized at less than 1 cm, 1 cm - 2cm and >2 cm respectively. This failure to identify a significant proportion of smaller tumors is indicative of the fact that a positive auditory brainstem response result is dependent upon a mass effect upon the cochlear nerve, and has led to the reservation of the technique as a second-line investigation. (Schmidt et al. 2001).

Despite its dubious sensitivity, the ABR provides a lot of information on the physiology of the auditory nerve and, therefore, is useful to establish an auditory prognosis in the case of possible surgical treatment with hearing preservation (the latency of the V-wave and the I-V interval value would be correlated with hearing conservation). On the other hand, the presence of abnormalities in the latencies of the ABR on the contralateral side of the tumor could suggest a distortion of the brainstem that would be associated with a poor postoperative facial function. (Matthies and Samii 1997, Di Stadio et al. 2018).

Vestibular Diagnostics

The presence of a VS usually leads to impairment of the afferent vestibular pathways as well as damage to the labyrinthine structures. For the diagnosis as well as post-therapeutic follow-up of patients with VS, vestibular diagnostics play a key role. Investigation of vestibular function requires the application of a vestibular stimulus and the observation of the reflexive eye movements (Vestibular Ocular Reflex – VOR), either using the naked eye, Frenzel Glasses, or by videonystagmography. Current tests include the head impulse test, calorics, rotational chair testing, Vestibular Evoked Myogenic Potential Cervical, Vestibular Evoked Myogenic Potential Ocular. The specificity and sensitivity of these tests concerning unilateral and bilateral vestibular dysfunction differ. Much of the current literature supports the use of caloric testing in the assessment of unilateral vestibular dysfunction. As such it is considered the clinical "gold standard." (Fife et al. 2000).

Caloric Reflex Testing

Caloric reflex testing with eye movement recording has long been considered the clinical gold standard for investigation of vestibular hypofunction due to VS. Temperature-induced convection currents lead to gravity-induced endolymph movement and consequent nystagmus is still considered the primary underlying physiological event. (Stahle 1990).

The Fitzgerald and Hallpike bi-thermal caloric test, devised in 1942, which employs two water temperatures alternately (30°C and 44°C), has demonstrated higher sensitivity than mono-thermal testing assessing that the stimulus should be small to restrict excitation to the lateral canal and a hot and cold stimuli of close equidistance to body temperature is enough to identify small changes in the reflex mechanisms. (Harvey, Wood and Feroah 1997).

The sensitivity of calorics in identifying vestibular hypofunction in unilateral VS has ranged from 50-100% depending on tumor size. (Haapaniemi et al. 2000). Some drawbacks have limited the use of this test: the incomplete ear irrigation can produce diminished responses, calorics may induce nausea, vertigo, and migraine. Testing may not be possible on those with tympanic membrane perforation, or recent ear surgery, anyway, as it is considered the "clinical gold standard" studies assessing new vestibular tests are compared to calorics.

Head Impulse Testing

Head impulse testing (HIT) is an established measure of the high-velocity VOR. Examiner driven head rotation to one side induces endolymph movement, which deforms the cupula of both lateral semicircular canals. This induces both a contralateral inhibitory and an ipsilateral excitatory response along the vestibular nerve to the vestibular nuclei. In patients with a unilateral deficit, the diminished response from the ipsilateral affected side and saturation of the contralateral inhibitory response leads to a failure of the VOR and a catchup saccade, this last can be recorded using video-oculography and quantified in terms of gain.

The low sensitivity (34-39%) and high specificity (100%) of HIT may be a consequence of how it is quantified. (Weber et al. 2008, MacDougall et al. 2009).

Rotational Chair Testing

In this test, patients are secured in a chair designed to rotate at set frequencies. The stimuli induce endolymph flow and cupula displacement activating the VOR. Rotary chair testing stimulates both vestibular labyrinths simultaneously; as most VS are unilateral they are often better evaluated by tests that stimulate each side separately. (Fife et al. 2000).

Vestibular Evoked Myogenic Potentials

Vestibular-evoked myogenic potentials (VEMP) are inhibitory electrical potentials generated after a sound stimulus (clicks or pure tones), either clicks or high-frequency tones are conveyed to the vestibular system by air or bone conduction. This activates the vestibular system, inducing a reproducible myogenic response in the cervical, and extra-ocular muscles. The cervical vestibular evoked myogenic potential (cVEMP) and ocular vestibular evoked myogenic responses (oVEMP) may be distinguished by recording activity in either the sternocleidomastoid (SCM) or oculomotor muscles. It is now generally considered that cVEMP is of saccular origin and oVEMP of utricular origin. (Rauch 2006).

As the cVEMP is an inhibitory response the SCM muscle has to be active; to achieve this, the subject either raises their head off the pillow or turns their head to the non-test side. In contrast, oVEMP is an excitatory response and the eyes may be at rest during recording, but this response appears to be best recorded from the inferior oblique muscle with the subject looking upwards. VEMP dysfunction can be characterized by the presence or absence of a response, calculating the asymmetry ratio between the amplitude of potentials generated from both ears (analogous to canal paresis in caloric testing), or comparing response latency. (Kantner and Gurkov 2012, Piras et al. 2013).

There are few studies of VEMPs in patients with VS. Abnormal oVEMP has been reported in 70% to 80% of VS patients, as few as 37.5% of patients in one study. (Piras et al. 2013).

Chiarovano et al., in their study, identified abnormal oVEMP in nine of 12 patients, but only 50% had an abnormal cVEMP; there was a weak correlation with canal paresis. However, despite this, the mean waveform latencies were not significantly different from normal. This suggests that while oVEMP is potentially superior for monitoring VS, it still has limited usefulness. (Chiarovano et al. 2011).

Imaging Diagnostics

Imaging diagnosis of the cerebellopontine angle (CPA) and the internal auditory canal (IAC) has evolved remarkably in the last decades.

Plain X-ray imaging was used at the beginning of the 20th century. The major problem was its inability to exactly depict soft tissues. Moreover, the radiolucency of a VS hardly differs from that of the surrounding brain tissue. As a consequence, the tumor often cannot be distinguished. On the other hand, bony structures can be depicted quite well using plain X-ray techniques. Per orbital view roentgenograms may reveal the presence of widening or funneling of the internal auditory canal. (Stemvers 1928).

The problem was, however, that this canal is not always widened in VS patients, particularly when the tumor has a prominent extrameatal localization. Moreover, it might be problematic to reliably assess abnormalities in the shape of the IAC since anatomical variations in its size and shape may occur.

The use of contrast substances was developed to improve the visualization of space-occupying lesions. For this purpose, several radiopaque substances, as well as just air, have been used. Intrathecal administration via a lumbar or suboccipital puncture was needed to allow the contrast material to reach the cerebellopontine cisternae. From the patient's perspective, this was an unpleasant and uncomfortable experience, and it was not without risk. Considerable progress was achieved with the introduction of computerized tomography (CT) in the 1970s. (Meijenhorst et al. 1984). CT scanning allows better visualization of the bony structures of the skull base, and minor differences in radiolucency of soft tissues which can be magnified. With the combination of CT and intrathecal administration of contrast substances (CT cisternography), nearly 100% sensitivity could be achieved to rule out CPA tumors. (Van et al. 1986, Scorpecci et al. 2018). However, contrast cisternography has remained a risky and invasive procedure as well as tumors less than 15 mm were often missed or unreliably diagnosed in the form of false-positives. (Cueva 2004).

Magnetic Resonance

In the mid-80's decade, CT has been displaced by magnetic resonance (MR), it has revolutionized the diagnosis of cerebellopontine angle pathology showing to be a more effective imaging modality than the CT scan in ruling out VS.

No contrast is required in the cerebellopontine cistern and no potentially harmful X-rays are needed, the procedure can be repeated as long as needed, and the size and shape of the tumor can be accurately assessed with MRI. (Singh et al. 2014).

MRI with contrast material, in particular, has greatly increased the sensitivity of the imaging and improved detection rates of VS. Today it is considered the clinical gold standard imaging technique for the diagnosis of this tumor as well as allows for monitoring of tumor growth. (Zamani 2000).

In the MRI the VS typically appears, except in unusual circumstances, as lobular almost spherical isodense lesion without contrast. With contrast (generally a T1-weighted scan before and after the introduction of Gadolinium contrast), they are seen as augmenting masses of greatly varying size occupying the cerebellopontine angle without dural tails. Distortion of the brainstem occurs without infiltration or edema and the tumor displays high contrast enhancement after gadolinium intravenous injection. The tumor may show variation in enhancement patterns depending on the size of the tumor and histological composition: homogenous (50 to 60%) composed predominantly of Antoni A type cells, heterogeneous (30 to 40%) have mixed Antonie A and Antonie B cells, or cystic (5 to 15%). (Bonneville, Savatovsky and Chiras 2007).

VSs do not have a footplate on the dura which is what usually distinguishes them from meningiomas. Small tumors may be entirely contained within the canal, and the smallest may measure only a few millimeters. Rarely, hemorrhage occurs within an acoustic tumor. (Chou, Sampath and Brem 1998).

Three-dimensional, fast spin-echo, heavily T2-weighted sequences (axial and crown planes) such as FIESTA (fast imaging employing steady-state acquisition) and CISS (constructive interference in steady-state) can also provide additional information regarding the branch of origin of the tumor, tumor volume and other CPA cranial nerves, including the facial nerve. (Thomas et al. 2008). However, imaging never replaces the need for intra-operative observation and neurophysiologic monitoring because the facial nerve is often close to the tumor capsule.

Conclusion

At present, MRI, audiometry, and vestibular diagnostics are the mainstays of the clinical workup for patients with SV. So, when pure-tone audiometry detects asymmetrical sensorineural hearing loss (which can be confirmed too by speech audiometry and ABR test), electronystagmography reveals vestibular dysfunction, and/or the patient reports asymmetrical tinnitus, a magnetic resonance imaging examination will follow to exclude the presence of VS. Currently, T1-weighted MRI using gadolinium-based contrast is the gold standard in the diagnostic workup of these patients.

REFERENCES

Angeli S., Jackson C. (1997) Neurotological evaluation. *Acoustic tumors diagnosis and management,* 85-91.

Bakkouri, WE, RE Kania, JP Guichard, G Lot, P Herman and PT Huy. 2009. "Conservative management of 386 cases of unilateral vestibular schwannoma: tumor growth and consequences for treatment." *J Neurosurg* 110:662-669.

Bonneville, F, J Savatovsky and J Chiras. 2007. "Imaging of cerebellopontine anglelesions: an update. Part 1: enhancing extra-axial lesions." *Eur Radiol* 17:2472-2482.

Chiarovano, E, F Zamith, PP Vidal and C de Waele. 2011. "Ocular and cervical VEMPs: a study of 74 patients suffering from peripheral vestibular disorders." *Clin Neurophysiol* 122(8):1650-1659.

Chou, D, P Sampath and H Brem. 1998. "Hemorrhagic vestibular schwannoma: an unusual clinical entity. Case report." *Neurosurg Focus* 5:e9.

Clark, JG. 1981. "Uses and abuses of hearing loss classification." *ASHA* 23:493-500.

Cueva, RA. 2004. "Auditory brainstem response versus magnetic resonance imaging for the evaluation of asymmetric sensorineural hearing loss." *Laryngoscope* 114:1686-1692.

Dandy, WE. 1918. "Ventriculography Following the Injection of Air into the Cerebral Ventricles." *Ann Surg* 68:5-11.

De Stefano A, Kulamarva G, Dispenza F. (2012) Malignant paroxysmal positional vertigo. *Auris Nasus Larynx;* 39:378-382.

Dispenza F., Cappello F, Kulamarva G, De Stefano A. (2015) The discovery of the stapes. *Acta Otorhinolaryngol Ital.* 33:357-359.

Dispenza F., Battaglia AM, Salvago P., Martines F. (2018) Determinants of failure in the reconstruction of the tympanic membrane: a case-control study. *Iranian Journal Otorhinolaryngology,* 30:341-346.

Di Stadio, A., Dipietro, L., Toffano, R., Burgio, F., De Lucia, A., Ippolito, V., Garofalo, S., Ricci, G., Martines, F., Trabalzini, F., Della Volpe, A. (2018) Working memory function in children with single side deafness using a bone-anchored hearing implant: A case-control study. *Audiology and Neurotology,* 23 (4), pp. 238-244.

Driscoll, CLW. (2000) Vestibular schwannoma (acoustic neuroma). *Tumors of the ear and temporal bone*, 172-218.

Fife, TD, RJ Tusa, JM Furman, DS Zee, E Frohman, RW Baloh, T Hain, J Goebel, J Demer and L Eviatar. 2000. "Assessment: vestibular testing techniques in adults and children: report of the Therapeutics and Technology Assessment Subcommittee of the American Academy of Neurology." *Neurology* 55(10):1431-1441.

Foley, RW, S Shirazi, RM Maweni, K Walsh, RM Walsh, M Javadpour and D Rawluk. 2017. "Signs and Symptoms of Acoustic Neuroma at Initial Presentation: An Exploratory Analysis." *Cureus 9*(11): e1846.

Fortnum, H, C O'Neill, R Taylor, R Lenthall, T Nikolopoulos, G Lightfoot, G O'Donoghue, S Mason, D Baguley, H Jones, and C Mulvaney. 2009. "The role of magnetic resonance imaging in the identification of suspected acoustic neuroma: a systematic review of clinical and cost effectiveness and natural history." *Health Technol Assess* 13:1-154.

Gouveris, HT, A Victor and WJ Mann. 2007. "Cochlear origin of early hearing loss in vestibular schwannoma." *Laryngoscope* 117:680-683.

Gardner, G and JH Robertson. 1988. "Hearing preservation in unilateral acoustic neuroma surgery." *Ann Otol Rhinol Laryngol* 97(1):55-66.

Haapaniemi, JJ, ET Laurikainen, R Johansson, T Rinne and M Varpula. 2000. "Audiovestibular findings and location of an acoustic neuroma." *Eur Arch Otorhinolaryngol* 257(5):237-241.

Harner, SG and ER Laws. 1981. "Diagnosis of acoustic neurinoma." *Neurosurgery* 9(4):373-379.

Harner, SG and ER Laws. 1983. "Clinical findings in patients with acoustic neuroma." *Mayo Clinic Proc* 58: 721-728.

Harvey, SA, DJ Wood and TR Feroah. 1997. "Relationship of the head impulse test and head-shake nystagmus in reference to caloric testing." *Am J Otol* 18(2):207-213.

Hentschel, M, M Scholte, S Steens, H Kunst and M Rovers. 2017. "The diagnostic accuracy of non-imaging screening protocols for vestibular schwannoma in patients with asymmetrical hearing loss and/or unilateral audiovestibular dysfunction: a diagnostic review and meta-analysis." *Clin Otolaryngol* 42(4):815-823.

Kentala, E and I Pyykko. 2001. "Clinical picture of vestibular schwannoma." *Auris Nasus Larynx* 28(1):15-22.

Katz J., Chasin M., English KM., Hood L. J., Tillery KL. (2015). *Handbook of clinical audiology*.

Kanzaki, J, M Tos, M Sanna and DA Moffat. 2003. "New and modified reporting system from the consensus meeting on systems for reporting results in vestibular schwannoma." *Otol Neurotol* 24:642-648.

Kantner, C and R Gurkov R. 2012. "Characteristics and clinical applications of ocular vestibular evoked myogenic potentials." *Hearing Res* 294(1-2):55-63.

MacDougall, HG, K Weber, LA McGarvie, G Halmagyi and I Curthoys. 2009. "The video head impulse test: diagnostic accuracy in peripheral vestibulopathy." *Neurology* 73(14):1134-1141.

Margolis, RH and GL Saly. 2008. "Asymmetric hearing loss: definition, validation, and prevalence." *Otol Neurotol* 29:422-431

Mathew, GD, GW Facer, KW Suh, OW Houser and PC O'Brien. 1978. "Symptoms, findings, and methods of diagnosis in patients with acoustic neuroma." *Laryngoscope* 88(12):1893-1903.

Matthies, C and M Samii. 1997. "Management of vestibular schwannomas (acoustic neuromas): The value of neurophysiology for evaluation and prediction of auditory function in 420 cases." *Neurosurgery* 40(5):919-930.

Matthies, C and M Samii. 1997. "Management of 1000 vestibular schwannomas (acoustic neuromas): clinical presentation." *Neurosurgery* 40(1):1-9.

Meijenhorst, GC, BA van der Lande, HH Baretta-Kooi HH, CR van der Kooi, AF Kroes and van Gasteren JH. 1984. "High-resolution CT and air CT cisternography in the diagnosis of acoustic neuromas." *Diagn Imaging Clin Med* 53(3):120-127.

Paul, BC and JT Roland. 2015. "An abnormal audiogram." *Jama* 313:85-86.

Paulraj, MP, K Subramaniam, SB Yaccob, AH Adom and CR Hema. 2015. "Auditory evoked potential response and hearing loss: a review." *Open Biomed Eng J* 9:17-24.

Piras, G, C Brandolini, A Castellucci and GC Modugno. 2013. "Ocular vestibular evoked myogenic potentials in patients with acoustic neuroma." *Eur Arch Otorhinolaryngol* 270(2):497-504.

Rauch, SD. 2006. "Vestibular evoked myogenic potentials." *Curr Opin Otolaryngol Head Neck Surg* 14(5):299-304.

Rogg, JM, SH Ahn, GA Tung, SE Reinert and G Noren. 2005. "Prevalence of hydrocephalus in 157 patients with vestibular schwannoma." *Neuroradiol* 47(5):344-351.

Roosli, C, FH Jr Linthicum, S Cureoglu and SN Merchant. 2012. "What is the site of origin of cochleovestibular schwannomas?" *Audiol Neuroto* 17:121-125.

Saliba, I, M Bergeron, G Martineau and M Chagnon. 2011. "Rule 3,000: a more reliable precursor to perceive vestibular schwannoma on MRI in screened asymmetric sensorineural hearing loss." *Eur Arch Otorhinolaryngol* 268:207-212.

Sauvaget, E, S Kici, R Kania, P Herman and PT Huy. 2005. "Sudden sensorineural hearing loss as a revealing symptom of vestibular schwannoma" *Acta Otolaryngol* 125(6):592-595.

Schmidt, RJ, RT Sataloff, J Newman, JR Spiegel and DL Myers. 2001. "The sensitivity of auditory brainstem response testing for the diagnosis of acoustic neuromas." *Arch Otolaryngol Head Neck Surg* 127(1):19-22.

Scorpecci, A., Massoud, M., Giannantonio, S., Zangari, P., Lucidi, D., Martines, F., Foligno, S., Di Felice, G., Minozzi, A., Luciani, M., Marsella, P. (2018) Otogenic lateral sinus thrombosis in children: proposal of an experience-based treatment flowchart. *European Archives of Oto-Rhino-Laryngology,* 275 (8), pp. 1971-1977.

Selesnick, SH, RK Jackler and LW Pitts. 1993. "The changing clinical presentation of acoustic tumors in the MRI era." *Laryngoscope.* 103:431-436.

Singh, K, MP Singh, C Thukral, K Rao, K Singh and A Singh. 2014. "Role of magnetic resonance imaging in evaluation of cerebellopontine angle schwannomas." *Indian J Otolaryngol Head Neck Surg* 67(1):21-27.

Stahle, J. 1990. "Controversies on the caloric response. From Barany's theory to studies in microgravity." *Acta Otolaryngol* 109(3-4):162-167.

Stangerup, SE, P Caye-Thomasen, M Tos and J Thomsen. 2006. "The natural history of vestibular schwannoma." *Otol Neurotol* 27:547-552.

Stemvers HW. (1928) *Röntgenologie des felsenbeines und des bitemporalen schädelbildes: mit besonderer berücksichtigung ihrer klinischen bedeutung* [*Roentgenology of the petrous bone and the bitemporal skull: with special consideration of its clinical significance.*].

Stucken, EZ, K Brown and SH Selesnick. 2012. "Clinical and diagnostic evaluation of acoustic neuromas." *Otolaryngol Clin North Am* 45(2):269-284.

Thomas, B, T Krishnamoorthy, HR Arvinda and CJ Kesavadas. 2008. "3D-CISS MRI in a purely intracanalicular cochlear schwannoma." *Neuroradiol* 35(5):305-307.

Van Dijk, JE, J Duijndam and K Graamans. 2000. "Acoustic neuroma: deterioration of speech discrimination related to thresholds in pure-tone audiometry." *Acta Otolaryngol* 120(5):627-632.

Van, SL, W Ampe, M Depondt and G D'Hont. 1986. "Role of air-CT-meato-cisternography in the diagnosis of acoustic neuroma." *Acta Otorhinolaryngol Belg* 40(4):644-657.

Von Kirschbaum, C and R Gürkov R. 2016. "Audiovestibular Function Deficits in Vestibular Schwannoma." *Biomed Res Int* 2016.

Weber, K, S Aw, M Todd, L McGarvie, I Curthoys and G Halmagyi. 2008. "Head impulse test in unilateral vestibular loss: Vestibulo-ocular reflex and catch-up saccades." *Neurology* 70(6):454-463.

West, N, H Sass, MN Møller, and P Cayé-Thomasen. 2018. "Facial nerve schwannomas presenting with vestibular dysfunction: a case series." *Acta Neurochir (Wien)* 160(12):2315-2319.

Zamani, AA. 2000. "Cerebellopontine angle tumors: role of magnetic resonance imaging." *Top Magn Reson Imaging* 11:98-107.

In: Vestibular Schwannoma
Editors: Francesco Dispenza et al.
ISBN: 978-1-53617-191-4

Chapter 3

NEUROFIBROMATOSIS TYPE 2

Tiziana Fragapane[1], Emanuela Salzano[1], Davide Vecchio[1] and Maria Piccione[1,2]

[1]Regional Reference Center for Rare Genetic and Chromosomal Diseases, A. O. Ospedali Riuniti "Villa Sofia-Cervello", Palermo, Italy

[2]Department of Sciences for the Promotion of Health and Maternal and Child Care "G. D'Alessandro", University of Palermo, Palermo, Italy

ABSTRACT

Neurofibromatosis type 2 (NF2) is a rare neurocutaneous disorder characterised by bilateral vestibular schwannomas associated with meningiomas, ependymomas and other cranial nerve and peripheral schwannomas. The clinical manifestations of NF2 show varying degrees of severity and age-related differences. Childhood presentation of NF2 also predicts a severe disease course. NF2 is genetically caused by germ-line mutations of the *NF2* gene located on 22q12.17. The *NF2* gene encodes a protein called merlin. Merlin associates with several transmembrane receptors and intracellular proteins serving as a tumor-suppressor. The diagnosis of NF2 is established based on clinical criteria, or combined molecular and clinical criteria. Specific genotype and phenotype correlations have been identified so far. Although significant progress in neurosurgery, radio-surgery and auditory rehabilitation have increased the treatment options for individuals with NF2, these show higher mortality rates than in the general population. Thus, tumour surveillance remains the cornerstone of NF2 patient management. Recent advances in the elucidation of the role of merlin have led to the development of biological targeted therapies.

Keywords: neurofibromatosis type 2, merlin, childhood NF2

Clinical Overview of Neurofibromatosis Type 2

Neurofibromatosis type 2 (NF2, OMIM 101000), first described in 1822 by the Scottish surgeon Wishart [1], is the second major form of neurofibromatosis, a group of neurogenetic disorders that share a predisposition to multiple tumours of the central and peripheral nervous systems, as well as other organs. While the incidence of Neurofibromatosis type 1 (NF1, OMIM 162200) is known to be 1 in every 2,500 to 3,000 births, the estimated incidence of NF2 is 1 per 25,000 to 33,000 live births [2]. Neurofibromatosis type 3 (NF3), also known as Schwannomatosis (OMIM 162091), is the least frequent form of neurofibromatosis with an estimated incidence of 1/40,000 – 1/70,000 [3]. NF2 is characterised by the development of bilateral vestibular schwannomas (VS) associated with multiple meningiomas, ependymomas, ocular and cutaneous abnormalities and peripheral neuropathy [4]. The clinical findings of NF2 are shown in Table 1.

Bilateral VS, also defined as acoustic neuromas, are the classic hallmark of NF2 and typically absent in Schwannomatosis [3]. VS are benign nerve sheath tumours and predominantly arise from the vestibular branches of the eighth cranial nerve. These present in patients usually by the age of 30 years with symptoms of deafness, tinnitus, balance dysfunction or facial nerve palsy [5]. VS may also cause severe neurological symptoms of brainstem compression, and life-threatening conditions such as massive intralesional haemorrhages [13]. Hearing loss in NF2 is a major morbidity. In contrast to other genetic causes of hypoacusis [14], no direct genotype-phenotype association has been established for hearing loss in NF2 [4]. Additionally, deafness in NF2 has an unpredictable onset and a variable progression, often not related to the tumour size and its growth rate. Thus, apart from the compressive effect of VS on the vestibulo-cochlear nerve, other pathogenetic mechanisms of hearing impairment have been hypothesised, such as cochlear aperture obstruction and the consequent increase of intralabyrinthine protein [15]. Although histologically similar to their sporadic counterparts, NF2-associated VS often appear multilobated (botryoid) and multifocal, instead of being ovoid and smooth like sporadic VS. Dewan et al. suggested that this multilobated appearance is due to a polyclonal origin of NF2-VS, arising from multiple, clonal tumours that undergo independent somatic "second hits" at *NF2* locus [16]. This finding may justify the worse treatment outcomes and the higher recurrence rates compared with sporadic VS.

Table 1. A broad spectrum of clinical findings can be associated with variable expressivity of NF2

Clinical features	Frequency of clinical feature
Bilateral vestibular schwannoma	90 – 95% [5, 6]
Unilateral vestibular schwannoma	18% [7]
Intracranial nonvestibular schwannoma	24 – 51% [6]
Intracranial meningioma	45 – 58% [5, 6]
Spinal tumour	63 – 90% [6, 8]
Ependymoma	18 – 58% [8, 9]
Peripheral nerve schwannoma	68% [5]
Subcutaneous tumour	43 – 48% [5, 10]
Skin plaques	41 – 48% [5, 10]
Intradermal tumour	27% [5]
Retinal hamartoma	6 – 22% [6]
Epiretinal membrane	12 – 40% [11]
Subcapsular cataract	60 – 81% [5, 11]
Peripheral neuropathy	6 – 66% [5, 12]

Schwannomas can form along the course of any other cranial or peripheral nerves, resulting different symptoms (pain, sensory loss, weakness) [4].

Meningiomas, often intracranial, occur in 15-20% of children and in half of adults with NF2 [7]. Although benign and slowly growing, meningiomas in NF2-patients are multiple and are assocatied with a 2.51-fold increase of relative risk of mortality [17]. In children with NF2, meningiomas are more likely to produce clinical symptoms related to their location (headache, seizures). Ependymomas, predominatly located in the intramedullary spinal cord, affect roughly 10% of children and 18-58% of adults [9]. These are WHO grade II and are usually asymptomatic, noted incidentally [4].

Cataracts associated with NF2 appear, on slit lamp examination, as opacities located in the posterior subcapsular, or peripheral cortical region of the lens. Cataracts are more common in childhood, and reduce visual acuity only in 10-20% of cases [6, 10]. Strabismus and nystagmus may occur due to peripheral vestibular dysfunction or eye involvement [18].

Cutaneous lesions include three types of skin tumours: skin plaques, subcutaneous tumours, and intradermal tumours. NF2 plaques are cutaneous schwannomas appearing as well defined, with a rough surface and with hyperpigmentation and excessive hair. Subcutaneous tumours are nodular schwannomas of peripheral nerves, occurring as well defined and usually spherical [7, 10]. Also, 'café au lait' macules are more prevalent than in the general population, but rarely reach the size or numbers seen in NF1 patients [10].

Peripheral neuropathy, either as mononeuropathy, or polineuropathy, can cause a progressive loss of sensory and motor function of peripheral nerves, typically distal extremities [12]. In childhood, it can present as a persistent facial palsy or hand/foot drop [7]. Initially attributed to the compressive effects of multiple tumourlets along the length of peripheral nerves, NF2-associated neuropathy often appears without tumours. Thus, *NF2* haploinsufficiency has been hypothesised as potentially pathogenetic [19].

The clinical presentation of NF2 is highly variable. Some individuals may have mosaic NF2, such as unilateral VS with ipsilateral tumours or segmental multiple schwannomas [20, 21]. Similarly to NF1, NF2 also shows age-dependent expression. In fact, despite its typical occurrence in young adulthood (age 20–30 years), approximately 18% of newly diagnosed patients with NF2 are younger than 15 years of age, and 9% are diagnosed before the age of 10 [7]. The most common initial signs of NF2 in childhood differ from adulhood, and consist in skin and ophthalmologic findings as well as neuropathy and intracranial meningiomas. These manifestations occur long before the typical hearing dysfunction [22]. Conversely, Ruggieri et al. described a congenital form of NF2, occurring in children before 1 year of age and characterized by (1) small, bilateral VS, usually asymptomatic and incidentally detected by MRI scans in the first months of life; (2) multiple NF2-related skin lesions; (3) lens opacities; (4) diffuse (asymptomatic) high signal lesions in the periventricular regions (e.g., cortical dysplasia); (5) no family history of NF2 [23].

GENETICS OF NF2

NF2 is inherited in an autosomal dominant manner and is caused by germ-line mutations of the *NF2* gene (locus 22q12.1) [5]. The *NF2* gene includes 17 exons spreading over 110 kb, and it encodes neurofibromin-2 (also called merlin or schwannomin) [24]. Both familial and sporadic cases have been equally reported. Furthermore, approximately 25-33% of sporadic cases are somatic mosaicisms, arising from mutations that take place after conception, resulting in two separate cell lineages [25]. Although the clinical expression of NF2 shows high interfamilial variability, in its classic form, there is a penetrance of approximately 100% by the age of 60 [26].

According to Knudson's two-hit hypothesis [27], the development of tumours in NF2 is caused by loss of function of the remaining normal copy of the gene, supported by findings of loss of herozygosity (LOH) in NF2 tumour samples [28]. Moreover, *NF2* somatic inactivation of both alleles has been documented in sporadic schwannomas (80%), in sporadic meningiomas (60%), and in sporadic ependymomas (5%) [29] . Interestingly, although somatic *NF2* are not common in human malignant cancers, they can occur in different types of cancers (e.g., mesothelioma, glioblastomas, breast and colorectal cancer, hepatobiliar and prostate cancers), affecting their therapeutic approach and prognosis [29].

Table 2. UK neurofibromatosis type 2 (NF2) Genetic Severity Score. Adapted from Halliday et al. [32]

Genetic severity	Subcategory	Clinical features	Definition
1 Tissue mosaic	1A	Presumed mosaicism	Meets clinical criteria for sporadic NF2 but not confirmed molecularly
	1B	Confirmed mosaicism	Mosaic NF2 confirmed molecularly with identical NF2 mutations detected in two or more separate tissue samples
2 Classic	2A	Mild NF2	Full or mosaic NF2 mutation identified in blood excluding those found in group 2B or 3: missense mutations; in-frame deletions and duplications; deletions involving the promoter region or exon 1; splice site mutations in exons 8–15; truncating mutations of exon 1; mosaicism in blood for mutations other than truncating mutations in exons 2–13
	2B	Moderate NF2	Full or mosaic NF2 mutation identified in blood including: splicing mutation involving exons 1–7; large deletion not including the promoter or exon 1; truncating mutations in exons 14–15; mosaic in blood for a truncating mutation in exons 2–13
3 Severe	3	Severe NF2	Full NF2 truncating mutation exons 2–13

Specific genotype-phenotype correlations in NF2 have been identified, based on the type of mutation, its position within the gene and its mosaic/constitutional state [30]. Generally, constitutional truncating *NF2* mutations (e.g., nonsense and frameshift mutations) are associated with severe phenotypes [30], whereas non-truncating mutations (e.g., missense mutations, and inframe or large deletions) lead to milder phenotypes [17]. Splicing *NF2* mutations are associated with variable disease severity [31]. Recently, Halliday et al. have proposed a Genetic Severity Score, that predicts clinical severity based on *NF2* mutation type (Table 2) [32]. In addition, complex chromosomal rearrangements involving chromosome 22 have also been reported to cause NF2. In particular, the ring chromosome 22 can cause the disruption of the *NF2* gene, leading to a complex phenotype with NF2-related tumours and additional features, including dysmorphisms, intellectual disability and congenital anomalies [33, 34].

MOLECULAR BIOLOGY OF NF2/MERLIN

Merlin (moesin-ezrin-radixin-like protein) is a member of the ERM (ezrin, radixin, moesin) family of proteins having a common N-terminal domain (FERM domain) [35]. Two major isoforms are produced by the alternative splicing of exon 16 (Figure 1A) [24, 35]. It remains obscure if the two isoforms have different functions, as long as tumourigenic mutations always inactivate both isoforms.

Merlin contains three highly conserved interaction domains: a FERM domain in its N-terminus, an α-helical domain, and a C-terminal domain (Figure 1B). In contrast to the other ERM proteins, merlin lacks the actin-binding site located in the C-terminal domain, instead it only has the FERM domain that links plasma membrane receptors to the cortical actin cytoskeleton [35, 36].

In addition, merlin can adopt two different conformations, depending on post-translational modifications [37]. Specifically, when it is phosphorylated at Ser518 by either p 21-actived kinases (PAKs), or protein kinase A (PKA), merlin has an 'open' (inactive) conformation, as it is unable to negatively regulate cell growth. Conversely, dephosphorylation of Ser518, by myosin phosphatase MYPT1–PP1δ, allows merlin to assume a 'closed' head-to-tail conformation that is considered active as a tumour suppressor (Figure 2) [37, 38].

Similarly to other ERM proteins, merlin is predominantly localized at the cell membrane-cytoskeletal interface. Here, it acts as a scaffold protein, providing a crucial link between the extacellular enviroment and the intracellular signaling pathways, and thus controlling cell-to-cell adhesion, and cellular proliferation [39]. Specifically, merlin interacts with cell adhesion receptors (e.g., CD44, β-catenin, cadherin, β1 integrin), receptor tyrosine kinases (RKTs), and small GTPases (e.g., Ras, Rac1), leading to the downstream regulation of various mitogenic signalling pathways, such as the phosphoinositide-3 kinase (PI3K)/Akt pathway, and the mitogen-activated protein kinase (MAPK) via Raf-ERK pathway (Figure 3) [36, 40]. These oncogenic pathways are crucial for promotion of cell growth, protein translation, and cellular proliferation. Furthermore, merlin is found at the nucleus of mammalian cells where it regulates the hippo signaling pathway, that normally inhibits organ growth by activating cell apoptosis and suppressing cell division [36, 41].

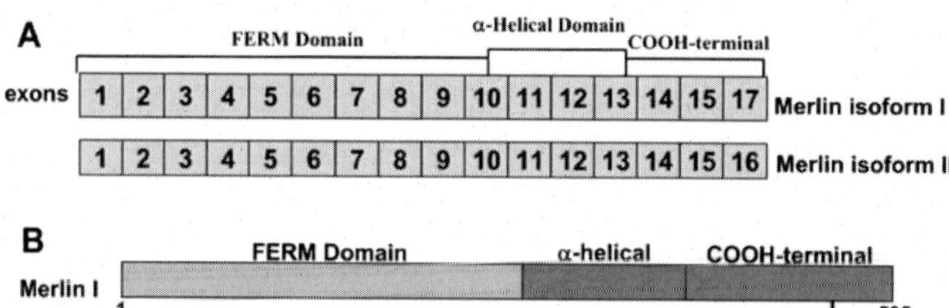

Figure 1. Exon organization and domain structure of merlin isoforms. (A) Merlin isoform 1 is coded by exons 1 to 15 and exon 17 and it includes 595 amino acids, while isoform 2 has 590 amino acid residues and results from the inclusion of alternatively spliced exon 16 that alters the C-terminal domain of the protein. (B) Domain organization of merlin isoform 1 is outlined. Adapted and modified from Stamenkovic and Yu [36].

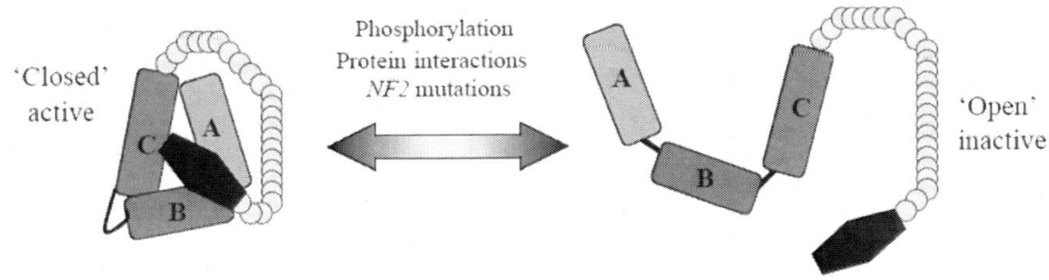

Figure 2. Merlin conformations are outlined. Adapted and modified from Sun et al. [37].

The *NF2* gene is expressed at high levels during embryonic development, as evidenced by the finding that complete inactivation of the mouse *NF2* gene results in embryonic lethality [42]. In adults, high expression is found in the peripheral nervous system and in neurons and astrocytes of the central nervous system, Schwann cells, meningeal cells, and lens [35].

Given its multifunctional role and its ubiquitous expression in human cells, it appears clear that merlin deficiency has a significant role in the pathogenesis of benign tumours in NF2 patients.

DIAGNOSIS OF NEUROFIBROMATOSIS TYPE 2

The diagnosis of NF2 is based on clinical evaluations. Different formal diagnostic criteria have been proposed [43, 44, 5, 45]. However, after the discovery of the *NF2* gene, it has become evident that *NF2* mutation testing might facilitate early diagnosis, in particular in childhood. Baser et al. developed a score system for the clinical diagnosis of NF2 that takes into account the age dependence of NF2 manifestations (Table 3) [46]. In addition, they included the mutational analysis of the NF2 gene as an essential part of diagnosis of NF2, especially in patients without a positive family history [46].

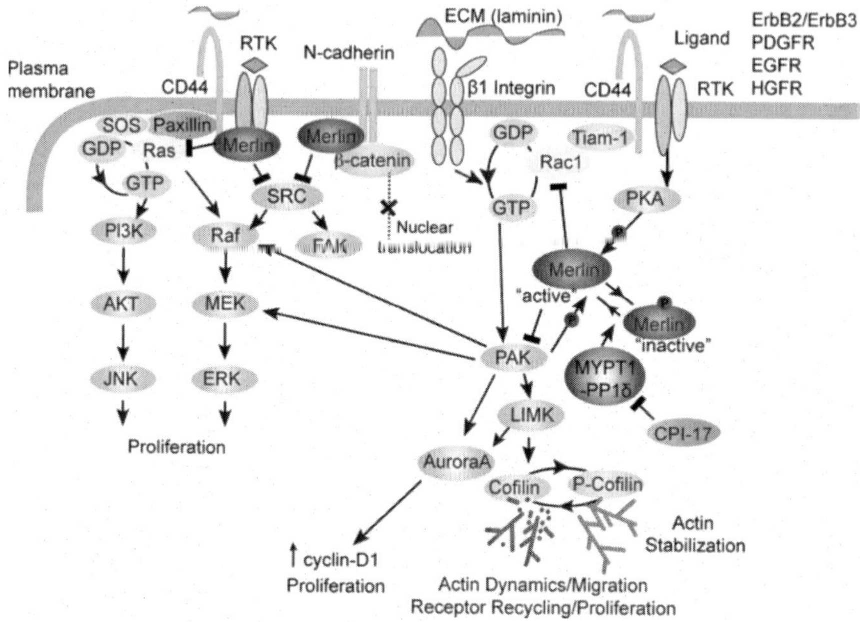

Figure 3. Merlin inhibits membrane receptors (CD44, RTKs) and RhoGTPase family signaling cascade. CD44 is a cell surface glycoprotein. In response to its ligand, the hyaluronan, a component of the extracellular matrix (ECM), CD44 promotes cell proliferation. When bound to NF2, CD44 is down-regulated. RKTs include different groups of receptor tyrosine kinases, namely ErbB receptors and Platelet derived growth factor receptor (PDGFR). The ErbB family, including EGFR, ErbB2, and ErbB3, are potent modulators of cell cycle progression. By binding the ErbB members, merlin inhibits cell growth. Similarly, merlin promotes PDGFR degradation, with a negative effect on the cell cycle progression. Among the RhoGTPases, Ras and Rac are well known to have significant ties to NF2. Indeed, merlin action on Ras signaling is indirect by blocking the assembly of Ras-complex, and inhibiting Ras-induced proliferations. Rac1, another member of RhoGTPase family, is capable of enhancing cyclin D1 expression, and thus promoting the G1 to S phase transition of the cell cycle. Merlin prevents this phenomenon by blocking the recruitment of Rac1 to the plasma membrane. Interestingly, a reciprocal interaction occurs in this pathway whereby Rac1 can activate PAK leading to merlin phosphorylation at Ser518 and its inhibition. Adapted and modified from Petrilli et al. [40].

A diagnosis of "definite NF2" is established if the total number of points is ≥ 6, or if the total number of points is 4 or 5 and a constitutional pathogenic NF2 mutation is found. Individuals with normal testing of NF2 in a blood sample should undergo genetic testing of tumour tissue to assess the presence of somatic mosaicism ("mosaic NF2"). In mutation-negative individuals, in both blood and tumour samples, a temporary diagnosis of "possible NF2" is made and a vigilant follow-up is required, as the disease evolves over time. Otherwise, in patients with a clinical score < 4, NF2 is "unlikely" and other disorders should be considered. This new set of diagnostic criteria shows a high specificity (100%) and sensitivity (79%), and thus allows clinicians to easily differentiate NF2 from the other neurofirbomatosis, in particular Schwannomatosis [46, 47].

Table 3. The Baser criteria for diagnosis of NF2. Adapted and modified from Baser et al. [46]

Feature	If present at or before the age of 30 years	If present after the age of 30 years
First-degree relative with NF2 diagnosed by these criteria	2	2
Unilateral vestibular schwannoma	2	1[a]
Second vestibular schwannoma	4	3[a]
One meningioma	2	1
Second meningioma (no additional points for more than two meningiomas)	2	1
Cutaneous schwannoma (one or more)	2	1
Cranial nerve tumour (excluding vestibular schwannoma) (one or more)	2	1
Mononeuropathy	2	1
Cataract (one or more)	2	0

The patient is given points as shown in the table.

[a] Points are not given for unilateral or second vestibular schwannoma if age at diagnosis is more than 70 years.

To date, standard sequencing analysis is able to detect 35-66% of pathogenic mutations, although adding deletion analysis (often by performing multiple ligation-dependent probe amplification, MLPA, and chromosomal microarray analysis, CMA), increases this proportion to about 90-95% in familial cases, and to 80-85% in sporadic cases [48]. Consideration should be given to cytogenetic tests (karyotype and fluorescence *in situ* hybridization, FISH) in patients with NF2-related tumours and intellectual disabilities, since ring chromosome 22 shows overlapping features [33, 34].

Management of Neurofibromatosis Type 2

Quality of life assessments are lower in both children and adults with NF2, due to hearing and balance impairment, facial disfigurement, and social isolation [49]. Overall survival rates, at 20 years after diagnosis, stand at 38% [50]. A young age at diagnosis and the presence of intracranial meningiomas are the most relevant predictors of poorer outcomes [17], in addition to specific genotypes [32]. Given the clinical complexity and the high morbidity and mortality rates of NF2, clinical management of NF2-patients consists in an early multidisciplinary surveillance program starting from diagnosis (Table 4) [51].

Table 4. Follow-up for confirmed cases of NF2. Adapted from Ardern-Holmes et al. [51]

	Frequency
Clinical examination	
• Audiologic examination	6 – 12 Months
• Skin examination	Annual
• Ocular examinations	Annual
• Neurologic examination	Annual
Neuroimaging (contrast enhanced MRI)	
• Brain with IAC	6 – 12 Months
• Spine	6 – 12 Months
Psychosocial support (assess employment/school/family functioning)	Annual
Genetic counseling	At diagnosis then at any stage

Audiological evaluations include pure tone audiometry, speech intelligibility assessment, and brainstem auditory evoked responses (BAERs) [52]. The best radiological investigation of intracranial and spinal tumours is through magnetic resonance imaging (MRI) with gadolinium contrast [4, 6]. Brain MRI scans should include high-resolution views of the internal auditory canal (IAC) in both axial and coronal planes. Surveillance spinal MRI scans are also recommended. Both brain and spinal MRI scans should be performed twice yearly following diagnosis, and then annually if there is no disease detected [51]. The timing of audiological evaluations and MRI scans depends on age and disease burden [50, 51].

Treatment of NF2-related tumours does not differ from standard treatment of their sporadic counterparts. However, in NF2 cases, therapy outcomes are consistently worse than in sporadic cases [50]. For VS, surgical removal and stereotactic radiosurgery are the current standard therapies. Different surgical approaches can be employed (sub-occipital, trans-labyrinthine). However, surgery is associated with lower rates of hearing preservation, and higher rates of disease recurrence and complications (facial nerve injury, lacrimal and swallowing dysfunction) in the treatment of NF2-related VS than in sporadic VS [16, 52]. This is likely due to the multifocal growth patterns and policlonality of NF2 tumorous lesions [16]. Stereotactic radiotherapy, usually with a γ–knife, has poorer outcomes for NF2 tumours, and it is also associated with the increased risk of malignant transformations [53]. Consequently, a reliable approach consists in watchful waiting, recommending surgical resection of VS only when they show rapid growth or symptomatic progression, and reserving radiation treatment for tumours that are not surgically accessible. In order to ensure a quality of life that is as good as possible, patients who are deaf with an intact cochlear nerve are candidates for auditory brainstem implantation [54]. Furthermore, regarding meningiomas, most of them do not require intervention. Surgery is the gold standard in symptomatic and rapidly enlarging tumours. Conversely, radiotherapy is recommended for malignant or multiple recurrent mengiomas, or those that are unresectable (e.g., involving the skull base, the cavernous sinuses, or the orbits) [55].

For ependymomas, total resection is indicated only when they are symptomatic, amd it is effective and curative [50].

Future Directions

The delineation of the NF2 biochemical signalling pathways has suggested strategies for developing targeted therapies [4, 50]. In the last few years, different categories of biological agents have been evaluated in clinical trials. For example, antagonists of the ErbB family (e.g., lapatinib, erlotinib), inhibitors of the Ras/Raf/Mek pathway (e.g., sorafenib, nilotinib), inhibitors of the Pi3K-Akt pathway (e.g., OSU3013, rapamycin), and antagonists of PDGF-R (e.g., sorafenib) [56]. The treatment that has shown the most promising results involves the use of Anti-VEGF antibodies. One of these is Bevazicumab, which has led to a reduction in vestibular schwannoma growth and the shrinking of tumours in some NF2 patients, improving their quality of life [56, 57]. However, this treatment is still at the trial stage.

References

[1] Wishart, J. H. (1822). Case of tumours in the skull, dura mater, and brain. *Edinburgh Med Surg J*, *18*, 393 - 397.

[2] Evans, D. G., Howard, E., Giblin, C., Clancy, T., Spencer, H., Huson, S. M. & Lalloo, F. (2010). Birth incidence and prevalence of tumor-prone syndromes: estimates from a UK family genetic register service. *Am J Med Genet A*, *152A*(2), 327 – 332.

[3] Koontz, N. A., Wiens, A. L., Agarwal, A., Hingtgen, C. M., Emerson, R. E. & Mosier, K. M. (2013). Schwannomatosis: the overlooked neurofibromatosis? *Am J Roentgenol*, *200*, W646 – W653.

[4] Asthagiri, A. R., Parry, D. M., Butman, J. A., Kim, H. J., Tsilou, E. T., Zhuang, Z. & Lonser, R. R. (2009). Neurofibromatosis type 2. *Lancet*, *373*(9679), 1974 - 1986.

[5] Evans, D. G., Huson, S. M., Donnai, D., Neary, W., Blair, V., Newton, V. & Harris, R. (1992). A clinical study of type 2 neurofibromatosis. *Q J Med*, *84*(304), 603 – 618.

[6] Mautner, V. F., Lindenau, M., Baser, M. E., Hazim, W., Tatagiba, M., Haase, W., Samii, M., Wais, R. & Pulst, S. M. (1996). The neuroimaging and clinical spectrum of neurofibromatosis 2. *Neurosurgery*, *38*, 880 – 885.

[7] Evans, D. G., Birch, J. M. & Ramsden, R. T. (1999). Paediatric presentation of type 2 neurofibromatosis. *Arch Dis Child*, *81*, 496 – 499.

[8] Dow, G., Biggs, N., Evans, G., Gillespie, J., Ramsden, R. & King, A. (2005). Spinal tumors in neurofibromatosis type 2. Is emerging knowledge of genotype predictive of natural history? *J Neurosurg Spine*, *2*, 574 – 579.

[9] Plotkin, S. R., O'Donnell, C. C., Curry, W. T., Bove, C. M., MacCollin, M. & Nunes, F. P. (2011). Spinal ependymomas in neurofibromatosis Type 2: a retrospective analysis of 55 patients. *J Neurosurg Spine*, *14*, 543 – 547.

[10] Mautner, V. F., Lindenau, M., Baser, M. E., Kluwe, L. & Gottschalk, J. (1997). Skin abnormalities in neurofibromatosis 2. *Arch Dermatol*, *133*, 1539 – 1543.

[11] Bosch, M. M., Boltshauser, E., Harpes, P. & Landau, K. (2006). Ophthalmologic findings and long-term course in patients with neurofibromatosis type 2. *Am J Ophthalmol*, *141*, 1068 – 1077.

[12] Sperfeld, A. D., Hein, C., Schroder, J. M., Ludolph, A. C. & Hanemann, C. O. (2002). Occurrence and characterization of peripheral nerve involvement in neurofibromatosis type 2. *Brain*, *125*, 996 – 1004.

[13] Gagliardo, C., Martines, F., Bencivinni, F., La Tona, G., Lo Casto, A. & Midiri, M. (2013). Intratumoral Haemorrhage Causing an Unusual

Clinical Presentation of a Vestibular Schwannoma. *The Neuroradiology Journal*, *26*, 30 – 34.

[14] Martines, F., Salvago, P., Bartolotta, C., Cocuzza, S., Fabiano, C., Ferrara, S., La Mattina, E., Mucia, M., Sammarco, P., Sireci, F. & Martines, E. (2015). A genotype-phenotype correlation in Sicilian patients with GJB2 biallelic mutations. *Eur Arch Otorhinolaryngol*, *272*(8), 1857 – 1865.

[15] Asthagiri, A. R., Vasquez, R. A., Butman, J. A., Wu, T., Morgan, K., Brewer, C. C., King, K., Zalewski, C., Kim, H. J. & Lonser, R. R. (2012) Mechanisms of Hearing loss in Neurofibromatosis Type 2. *PLoS ONE*, *7*(9), e46132.

[16] Dewan, R., Pemov, A., Kim, H. J., Morgan, K. L., Vasquez, R. A., Chittiboina, P., Wang, X., Chandrasekharappa, S. C., Ray-Chaudhury, A., Butman, J. A., Stewart, D. A. & Asthagiri, A. R. (2015). Evidence of polyclonality in neurofibromatosis type 2–associated multilobulated vestibular schwannomas. *Neuro-Oncology*, *17*(4), 566 – 573.

[17] Baser, M. E., Friedman, J. M., Aeschliman, D., Joe, H., Wallace, A. J., Ramsden, R. T. & Evans, D. G. (2002). Predictors of the Risk of Mortality in Neurofibromatosis 2. *Am. J. Hum. Genet*, *71*, 715 – 723.

[18] Feucht, M., Griffiths, B., Niemuller, I., Haase, W., Richard, G. & Mautner, V. F. (2008). Neurofibromatosis 2 leads to higher incidence of strabismological and neuro-ophthalmological disorders. *Acta Ophthalmol*, *86*, 882 – 886.

[19] Schulz, A., Zoch, A. & Morrison, H. (2014) A neuronal function of the tumor suppressor protein merlin. *Acta Neuropathologica Communications.*, *2*, 82.

[20] Ruggieri, M. & Huson, S. (2011) The clinical and diagnostic implications of mosaicism in the neurofibromatosis. *Neurology*, *56*, 1433 – 1443.

[21] Castellanos, E., Bielsa, I., Carrato, C., Rosas, I., Solanes, A., Hostalot, C., Amilibia, E., Prades, J., Roca-Ribas, F., Lázaro, C., Blanco, I. & Serra, E. (2015). Segmental neurofibromatosis type 2:

discriminating two hit from four hit in a patient presenting multiple schwannomas confined to one limb. *BMC Medical Genomics*, *8*, 2.

[22] Ruggieri, M., Praticò, A. D., Serra, A., Maiolino, L., Cocuzza, S., Di Mauro, P., Licciardello, L., Milone, P., Privitera, G., Belfiore, G., Di Pietro, M., Di Raimondo, F., Romano, A., Chiarenza, A., Muglia, M., Polizzi, A. & Evans, D. G. (2016). Childhood neurofibromatosis type 2 (NF2) and related disorders: from bench to bedside and biologically targeted therapies. *ACTA Otorhinolaryngologica Italica*, *36*, 345 – 367.

[23] Ruggieri, M., Gabriele, A. L., Polizzi, A., Salpietro, V., Nicita, F., Pavone, P., Platania, N., Milone, P., Distefano, A., Privitera, G., Belfiore, G., Granata, F., Caltabiano, R., Albanese, V., Pavone, L. & Quattrone, A. (2013) Natural history of neurofibromatosis type 2 with onset before the age of 1 year. *Neurogenetics*, *14*, 89 – 98.

[24] Rouleau, G. A., Merel, P., Lutchman, M., Sanson, M., Zucman, J., Marineau, C., Hoang-Xuan, K., Demczuk, S., Desmaze, C., Plougastel, B., Pulst, S. M., Lenoir, G., Bijlsma, E., Fashold, R., Dumanski, J., de Jong, P., Parry, D., Eldrige, R., Aurias, A., Delattre, O. & Thomas, G. (1993). Alteration in a new gene encoding a putative membrane-organizing protein causes neuro-fibromatosis type 2. *Nature*, *363*(6429), 515 – 521.

[25] Kluwe, L., Mautner, V., Heinrich, B., Dezube, R., Jacoby, L. B., Friedrich, R. E. & MacCollin, M. (2003) Molecular study of frequency of mosaicism in neurofibromatosis 2 patients with bilateral vestibularschwannomas. *J Med Genet*, *40*, 109 – 114.

[26] Evans, D. G., Huson, S. M., Donnai, D., Neary, W., Blair, V., Teare, D., Newton, V., Strachan, T., Ramsden, R. & Harris, R. (1992). A genetic study of type 2 neurofibromatosis in the United Kingdom. I. Prevalence, mutation rate, fitness, and confirmation of maternal transmission effect on severity. *J Med Genet*, *29*, 841 – 846.

[27] Knudson, A. G. Jr. (1971). Mutation and cancer: statistical study of retinoblastoma. *Proc Natl Acad Sci USA*, *68*, 820 – 823.

[28] Woods, R., Friedman, J. M., Evans, D. G., Baser, M. & Joe, H. (2003). Exploring the `2-Hit Hypothesis' in NF2: Tests of 2-Hit and

3 Hit models of vestibular schwannoma development. *Genet Epidemiol*, *24*, 265 – 272.

[29] Antinheimo, J., Sankila, R., Carpén, O., Pukkala, E., Sainio, M. & Jääskeläinen, J. (2000). Population-based analysis of sporadic and type 2 neurofibromatosis-associated meningiomas and schwannomas. *Neurology*, *54*(1), 71 – 76.

[30] Baser, M. E., Kuramoto, L., Joe, H., Friedman, J. M., Wallace, A. J., Gillespie, J. E., Ramsden, R. T. & Evans, D. G. (2004). Genotype-phenotype correlations for nervous system tumors in neurofibromatosis 2: a population-based study. *Am J Hum Genet*, *75*, 231 – 239.

[31] Baser, M. E., Kuramoto, L., Woods, R., Joe, H., Friedman, J. M., Wallace, A. J., Ramsden, R. T., Olschwang, S., Bijlsma, E., Kalamarides, M., Papi, L., Kato, R., Carroll, J., Lazaro, C., Joncourt, F., Parry, D. M., Rouleau, G. A. & Evans, D. G. (2005). The location of constitutional neurofibromatosis 2 (NF2) splice site mutations is associated with the severity of NF2. *J Med Genet*, *42*, 540 – 546.

[32] Halliday, D., Emmanouil, B., Pretorius, P., MacKeith, S., Painter, S., Tomkins, H., Evans, D. G. & Parry, A. (2017). Genetic Severity Score predicts clinical phenotype in NF2. *J Med Genet*, *54*, 657 – 664.

[33] Tsilchorozidou, T., Menko, F. H., Lalloo, F., Kidd, A., De Silva, R., Thomas, H., Smith, P., Malcolmson, A., Dore, J., Madan, K., Brown, A., Yovos, J. G., Tsaligopoulos, M., Vogiatzis, N., Baser, M. E., Wallace, A. J. & Evans, D. G. (2004). Constitutional rearrangements of chromosome 22 as a cause of neurofibromatosis 2. *J Med Genet*, *41*, 529 – 534.

[34] Lyons-Warren, A. M., Cheung, S. W. & Holder, L. J. Jr. (2017). Clinical Reasoning: A common cause for Phelan-McDermid syndrome and neurofibromatosis type 2. One ring to bind them. *American Academy of Neurology*, *89*(17), e205 – e209.

[35] Trofatter, J. A., MacCoiiin, M. M., Rutter, J. L., Murreil, J. R., Duyao, M. P., Parry, D. M., Eidridge, R., Kiey, N., Nlenon, A. G., Pulaski, K., Haase, V. H., Ambrose, C. M., Munroe, D., Bove, C., Haines, J. L., Martuza, R. L., MacDonald, M. E., Seizinger, B. R.,

Short, M. P., Buckler, A. J. & Gusella, J. F. (1993). A novel moesin-, ezrin-, radixin-like gene is a candidate for the neurofibromatosis 2 tumor suppressor. *Cell*, *72*, 791 – 800.

[36] Stamenkovic, I. & Yu, Q. (2010). Merlin, a "Magic" Linker Between the Extracellular Cues and Intracellular Signaling Pathways that Regulate Cell Motility, Proliferation, and Survival. *Curr Protein Pept Sci*, *11*(6), 471 – 484.

[37] Sun, C. X., Robb, V. A. & Gutmann, D. H. (2002). Protein 4.1 tumor suppressors: getting a FERM grip on growth regulation. *Journal of Cell Science*, *115*, 3991 – 4000.

[38] Surace, E. I., Haipek, C. A. & Gutmann, D. H. (2004). Effect of merlin phosphorylation on neurofibromatosis 2 (NF2) gene function. *Oncogene*, *23*, 580 – 587.

[39] Beltrami, S., Kim, R. & Gordon, J. (2013). Neurofibromatosis type 2 protein, NF2: an unconventional cell cycle regulator. *Anticancer Res*, *33*(1), 1 – 11.

[40] Petrilli, A. M. & Fernández-Valle, C. (2016). Role of Merlin/NF2 Inactivation in Tumor Biology. *Oncogene*, *35*(5), 537 – 548.

[41] Li, Y., Zhou, H., Li, F., Chan, S. W., Lin, Z., Wei, Z., Yang, Z., Guo, F., Lim, C. J., Xing, W., Shen, Y., Hong, W., Long, J. & Zhang, M. (2015). Angiomotin binding-induced activation of Merlin/NF2 in the Hippo pathway. *Cell Research*, *25*, 801 – 817.

[42] McClatchey, A. I., Saotome, I., Ramesh, V., Gusella, J. F. & Jacks, T. (1997). The NF2 tumor suppressor gene product is essential for extraembryonic development immediately prior to gastrulation. *Genes & development*, *11*(10), 1253 – 1265.

[43] National Institutes of Health Consensus Development Conference Statement. Neurofibromatosis. (1988). *Arch Neurol*, *45*, 575 – 578.

[44] Mulvihill, J. J., Parry, D. M., Sherman, J. L., Pikus, A., Kaiser-Kupfer, M. I. & Eldridge, R. (1990) Neurofibromatosis 1 (Recklinghausen Disease) and Neurofibromatosis 2 (Bilateral Acoustic Neurofibromatosis): An Update. *Ann Intern Med*, *113*, 39 – 52.

[45] Gutmann, D. H., Aylsworth, A., Carey, J. C., Korf, B., Marks, J., Pyeritz, R. E., Rubenstein, A. & Viskochil, D. (1997). The diagnostic evaluation and multidisciplinary management of neurofibromatosis 1 and neurofibromatosis 2. *JAMA.*, *278*(1), 51 – 57.

[46] Baser, M. E., Friedman, J. M., Joe, H., Shenton, A., Wallace, A. J., Ramsden, R. T. & Evans, D. G. (2011). Empirical development of improved diagnostic criteria for neurofibromatosis 2. *Genet Med*, *13*, 576 – 581.

[47] Baser, M. E., Friedman, J. M., Wallace, A. J., Ramsden, R. T. & Joe, H., Evans, D. G. (2002). Evaluation of clinical diagnostic criteria for neurofibromatosis 2. *Neurology*, *59*(11), 1759 – 1765.

[48] Evans, D. G. (2009). Neurofibromatosis type 2 (NF2): A clinical and molecular review. *Orphanet Journal of Rare Diseases*, *4*, 16.

[49] Neary, W. J., Hillier, V. F., Flute, T., Stephens, S. D., Ramsden, R. T. & Evans, D. G. (2010). The relationship between patients' perception of the effects of neurofibromatosis type 2 and the domains of the Short Form-36. *Clin. Otolaryngol*, *35*, 291 – 299.

[50] Blakeley, J. O., Evans, D. G., Adler, J., Brackmann, D., Chen, R., Ferner, R. E., Hanemann, C. O., Harris, G., Huson, S. M., Jacob, A., Kalamarides, M., Karajannis, M. A., Korf, B. R., Mautner, V. F., McClatchey, A. I., Miao, H., Plotkin, S. R., Slattery, W., Stemmer-Rachamimov, A. O., Welling, D. B., Wen, P. Y., Widemann, B., Hunter-Schaedle, K. & Giovannini, M. (2012). Consensus Recommendations for Current Treatments and Accelerating Clinical Trials for Patients with Neurofibromatosis Type 2. *Am J Med Genet A*, *158A*(1), 24 – 41.

[51] Ardern-Holmes, S., Fisher, G. & North, K. (2017). Neurofibromatosis Type 2: presentation, major complications, and management, with a focus on the pediatric age group. *Journal of Child Neurology*, *32*(1), 9 – 22.

[52] Plotkin, S. R., Ardern-Holmes, S. L., Barker, F. G., Blakeley, J. O., Evans, D. G., Ferner, R. E., Hadlock, T. A., Halpin, C. & REiNS International Collaboration. (2013). Hearing and facial function

outcomes for neurofibromatosis 2 clinical trials. *Neurology*, *81*, S25 – S32.

[53] Mathieu, D., Kondziolka, D., Flickinger, J. C., Niranjan, A., Williamson, R., Martin, J. J. & Lunsford, L. D. (2007). Stereotactic radiosurgery for vestibular schwannomas in patients with neurofibromatosis type 2: an analysis of tumor control, complications, and hearing preservation rates. *Neurosurgery*, *60*(3), 460 – 468.

[54] Lustig, L. R., Yeagle, J., Driscoll, C. L., Blevins, N., Francis, H. & Niparko, J. K. (2006) Cochlear implantation in patients with neurofibromatosis type 2 and bilateral vestibular schwannoma. *Otol Neurotol*, *27*, 512 – 518.

[55] Goldsmith, B. & McDermott, M. W. (2006). Meningioma. *Neurosurg Clin N Am*, *17*, 111 –120.

[56] Blakeley, J. O. & Plotkin, S. R. (2016). Therapeutic advances for the tumors associated with neurofibromatosis type 1, type 2, and schwannomatosis. *Neuro-Oncology*, *18*(5), 624 – 638.

[57] Plotkin, S. R., Merker, V. L., Halpin, C., Jennings, D., McKenna, M. J., Harris, G. J. & Barker, F. G. (2012). Bevacizumab for progressive vestibular schwannoma in neurofibromatosis type 2: a retrospective review of 31 patients. *Otol Neurotol*, *33*(6), 1046 – 1052.

In: Vestibular Schwannoma
Editors: Francesco Dispenza et al.
ISBN: 978-1-53617-191-4

Chapter 4

IMAGING OF VESTIBULAR SCHWANNOMA

Paola Feraco[1,2], MD, Silvia Piccinini[3], MD, Giuseppe Salvaggio[4], MD and Cesare Gagliardo[4,*], MD, PhD

[1]Department of Radiology, Ospedale S. Chiara, Azienda Provinciale per i Servizi Sanitari, Trento, Italy
[2]Department of Specialized, Diagnostic and Experimental Medicine (DIMES), University of Bologna, Bologna, Italy
[3]Department of Neuroradiology, Azienda Ospedaliero-Universitaria di Modena, Modena, Italy
[4]Section of Radiological Sciences - Department of Biomedicine, Neuroscience and Advanced Diagnostic, University of Palermo, Palermo, Italy

ABSTRACT

Lesions of the cerebellopontine angle and internal auditory canal are a frequent finding in neuroradiological examinations and their detection may represent a diagnostic challenge. Among these lesions, vestibular

* Corresponding Author's Email: cesare.gagliardo@gmail.com,

schwannomas and meningiomas are certainly the most frequent and account for up to 90% of all cerebellopontine angle tumours. The remaining ones are a group of lesions arising from the different structures found in these anatomical regions such as haemangiomas, lipomas, lymphomas, facial nerve tumours, and aneurysms. This chapter will introduce this topic focusing on a practical coverage of the typical and atypical neuroradiological signs that will drive towards the most correct differential diagnosis checklist. High-quality neuroradiological images will support the reader for an optimal learning experience.

1. Imaging Protocol of Cerebellopontine Angle and Internal Auditory Canal Lesions

Imaging techniques have historically supported the study of the auditory system which always required dedicated and optimized protocols to ensure a good visualization of its peculiar anatomy and related pathology. Computerized Tomography (CT) and Magnetic Resonance Imaging (MRI) are certainly the most used imaging modalities to investigate the cerebellopontine angle (CPA) and internal auditory canal (IAC). Lesions in the CPA or in the IAC are frequent and represent 6% – 10% of all intracranial tumors. Vestibular schwannomas and meningiomas are the two most frequent and account for approximately 85% – 90% of all CPA tumors [7-8]. The other 10% – 15% represents a group of lesions arising from the different structures found in these anatomical regions. These lesions are not easily differentiated based on clinical symptoms and physical examination and their detection is a diagnostic challenge. Asymmetric sensorineural hearing loss (aSNHL) is the most common symptom associated with Vestibular Schwannoma (VS). The diagnostic study with the greatest sensitivity and specificity in the evaluation aSNHL is MRI that is the method of choice for detection, staging and follow-ups of VSs.

CT is the primary imaging modality for evaluating the osseous components of the temporal bone region [1-2]. Multi-detector CT (MDCT) imaging protocols for temporal bone region are typically based on sub-millimetric slice thickness isotropic datasets which enable multiplanar reconstructions (MPR) for an optimal evaluation of the region of interest. All temporal bone examinations should be reconstructed using a bone algorithm and each side should be separately reconstructed using a magnified small field of view (FOV). Reconstruction of the posterior fossa using soft-tissue algorithm with a wider FOV is recommended. Intravenous (i.v.) administration of contrast medium is usually not indicated for CT temporal bone imaging in favor of an MRI study.

MRI is the primary imaging modality for evaluating the non-osseous components of the temporal bone region [3-4]. A high field strength MRI scanner (1.5 – 3.0 Tesla field strength) is typically used together with a phased array head coil. The use of dedicated surface coils can improve the signal-to-noise ratio at the cost of a lower depth and reduced FOV. To ensure a good visualization of the peculiar anatomy and related pathology of this region a small FOV is used and slice thickness should not exceed 3 mm with no interslice gap. A typical MRI protocol consists of the following sequences: axial T2-weighted (T2-w) Fluid Attenuated Inversion Recovery (FLAIR), axial and coronal T1-weighted (T1-w) Spin Echo (SE) or Turbo Spin Echo (TSE) (repeated after i.v. administration of paramagnetic contrast agent) and axial thin-slice (≤1mm) heavily T2-weighted 3D fast GRadient Echo (GRE). The whole brain T2-w FLAIR sequence, is generally used as an overview sequence to exclude other brain pathologies. The thin-slice heavily T2-w 3D fast GRE sequence, is particularly dependent on high gradient amplitude and slew rates and has a cisternographic effect showing very high contrast between liquor and surrounding structures (nerves, vessels, and bone). Even if each vendor uses a different name, nowadays the most commonly used 3D fast GRE pulse sequences are the 3D Constructive Interference In Steady-State (3D-CISS) [5]. These sequences are named Fast Imaging Employing Steady-state Acquisition (FIESTA) by General Electric Healthcare, true Fast Imaging with Steady-state Precession (FISP) by Siemens, Balanced Fast Field Echo (BFFE) by Philips and true Steady-State Free Precession (SSFP) by Toshiba. Whatever the vendor of the MRI scanner, the acquired 3D-CISS images can be re-formatted in arbitrary orientation because of the sub-millimetric isotropic resolution. It is suitable for exact tumor volumetry and for preoperative assessment of the tumor in relation to brainstem, fundus, vessels and nerves. To complete the examination, a T1-w 3D-TSE sequence is scanned. This high-resolution T1-w sequence is repeated after i.v. administration of paramagnetic contrast agent to improve the detection of very small tumors or for an optimal postoperative evaluation (i.e., differentiation between scars and residual tumor tissue or recurrences) [9-12]. A whole-brain Diffusion-Weighted Imaging (DWI) sequence can be optionally performed to exclude/confirm acute ischemia or to further characterize a CPA/IAC lesion (i.e.: arachnoid cyst vs epidermoid cyst). In patients in whom a cholesteatoma is suspected, DWI sequences have been shown to be specifically useful [6].

2. Vestibular Schwannoma

Acoustic neuroma, also known as vestibular schwannoma (VS) is the most frequent tumour in the CPA (70 - 80% of all CPA masses). It arises from the Schwann cells that wrap the vestibulocochlear nerve at glial-Schwann cell junction (Obersteiner-Redlich zone). VSs are usually unilateral, not hereditary and occur sporadically; bilateral vestibular schwannomas are usually associated with a genetic disorder (neurofibromatosis type 2, NF2).

Most VSs (up to 90%) develop from the inferior vestibular nerve in the IAC where they grow slowly (Figure 1). A minority of VSs are purely extracanalicular, merely abutting the porus acusticus, (20%) while rarely small tumors may be confined to the labyrinth.

At On imaging, VS classically presents as a solid nodular mass with intracanalicular component that often results in widening of the porus acusticus (Figure 2). At CT, schwannomas are usually isodense and enhance after contrast administration. On MRI, they show T1 isointensity and T2 high signal intensity (Figure 3a and 3b), but appear as a hypointense filling defect on T2-w high-resolution MR cisternography (3D CISS sequences) (Figure 3c).

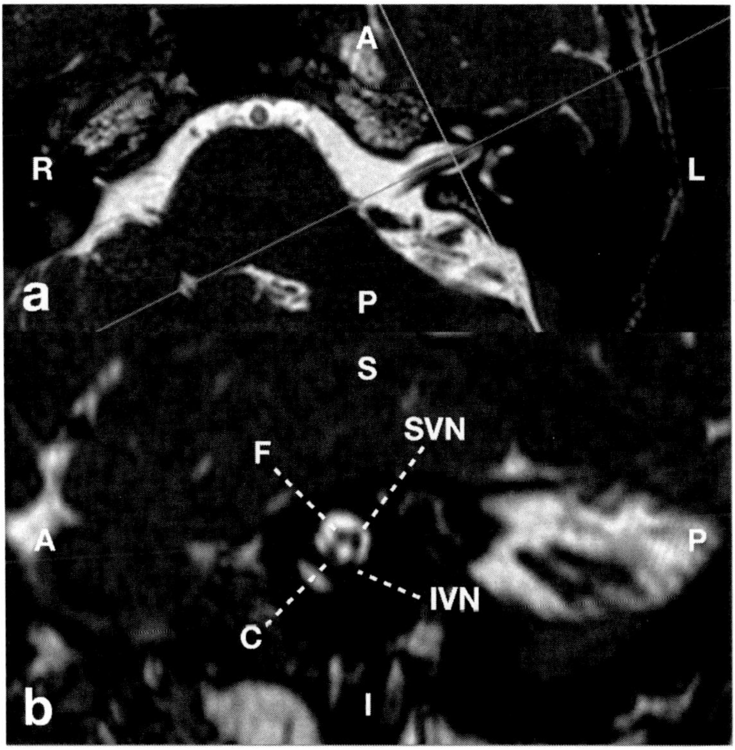

Figure 1. 3D CISS passing through the left internal auditory channel (IAC) showing the intracisternal tract of the 7th (anterior) and 8th (posterior) cranial nerves (upper row); superimposed DICOM references lines shows the correct oblique orientation of a MultiPlanar Reconstruction (MPR) to evaluate the internal auditory channel tracts: the resulting MPR plane (bottom row) shows the typical four black dots into the IAC: the facial nerve (F) is in an anterior-superior location, the cochlear nerve (C) is in an anterior-inferior location, the superior and the inferior vestibular nerves (SVN and IVN respectively) are located posteriorly. A: anterior; P: posterior; S: superior; I: inferior; R: right; L: left.

The 8th cranial nerve is surrounded by cerebrospinal fluid (CSF) which provides a natural contrast for MRI. Therefore, any internal acoustic meatus mass will squeeze the adjacent CSF away resulting into a hypointense area on T2-w sequences.

VS enhances strongly on T1-w sequences scanned after i.v. administration of paramagnetic contrast agent as result of the impaired vascular barrier from the active and untidy angiogenesis of the tumor (Figure 3d).

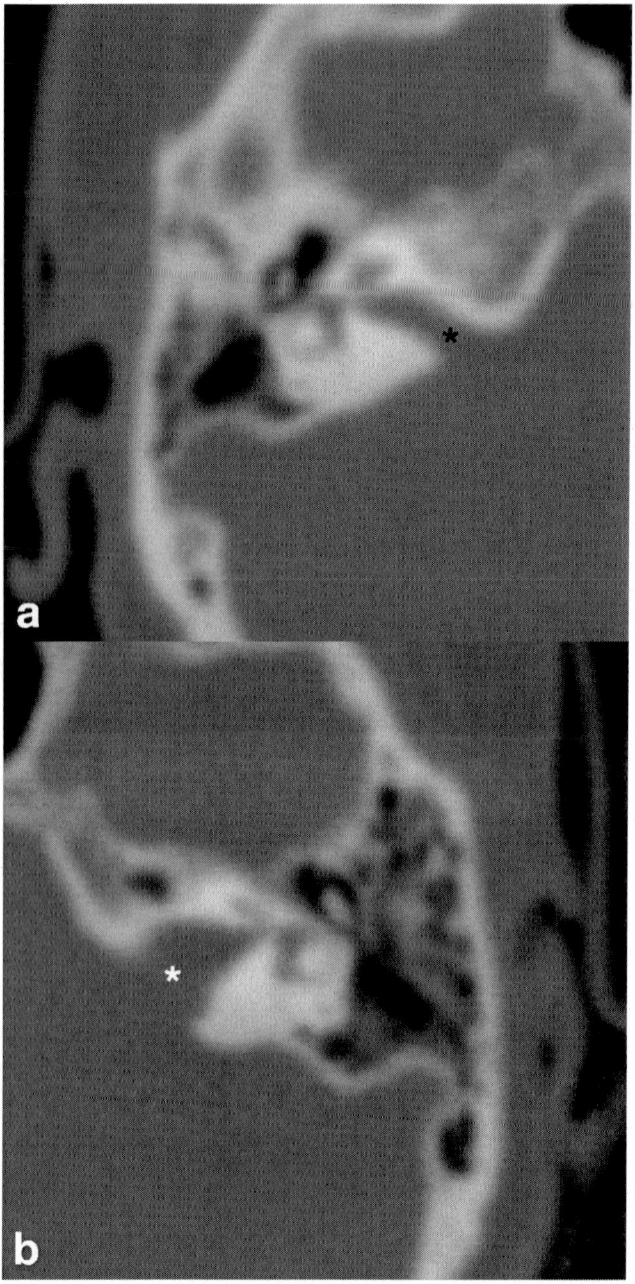

Figure 2. CT scan (bone window) demonstrate a widening of the left porus acusticus (white asterisk in b) in a patient with a giant vestibular schwannoma. Right porus acusticus is normal (black asterisk in a).

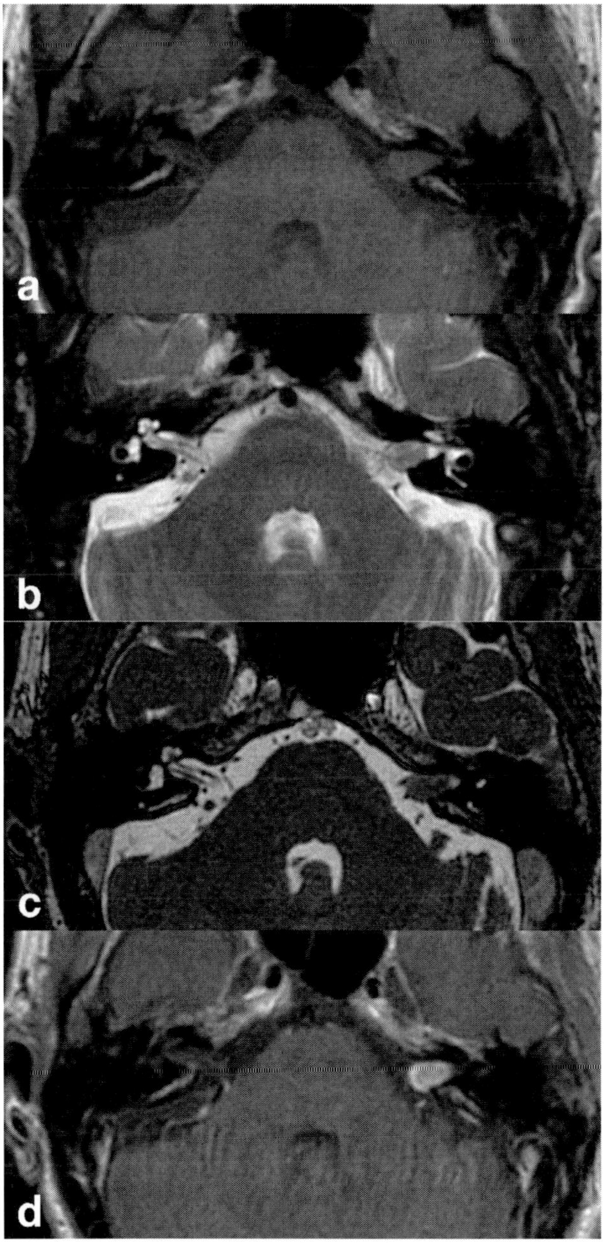

Figure 3. Typical neuroradiological findings of a small intracanalicular vestibular schwannomas. Solid components of the tumor show T1 isointensity (a) and T2 high signal intensity (b), but appear as a hypointense mass on 3D CISS (c). Intravenous contrast agent administration results in a homogeneous contrast enhancement (d).

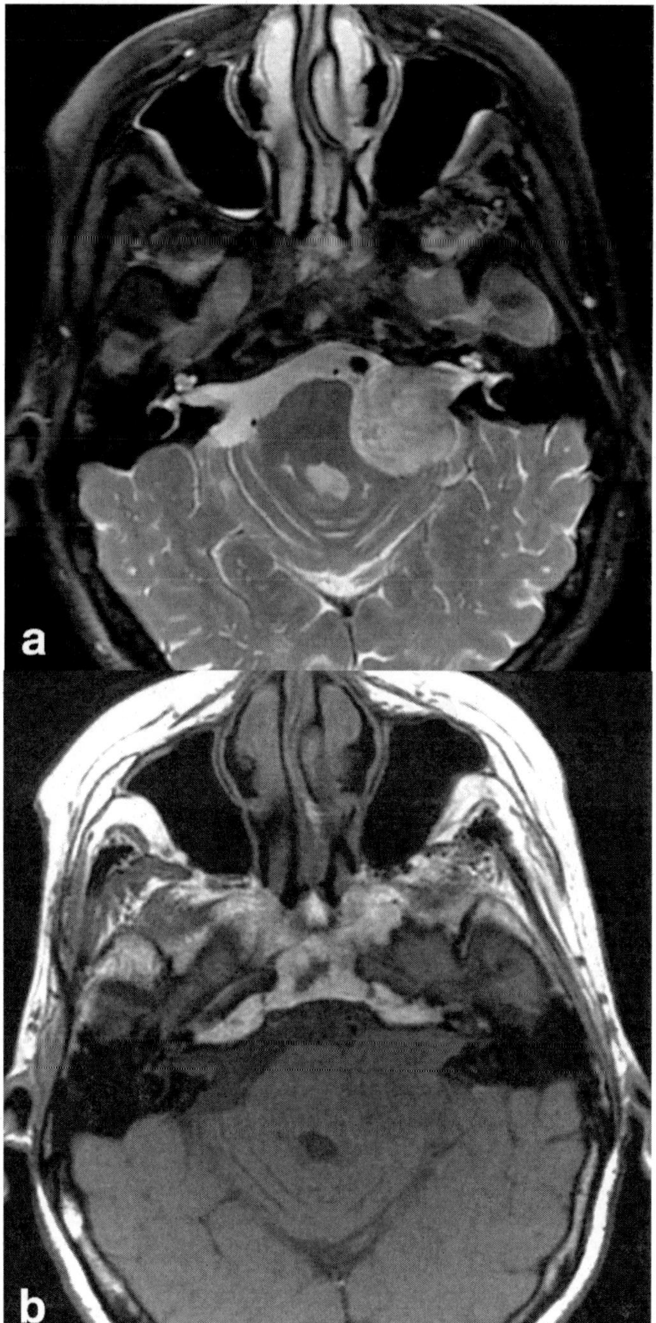

Figure 4. (Continued).

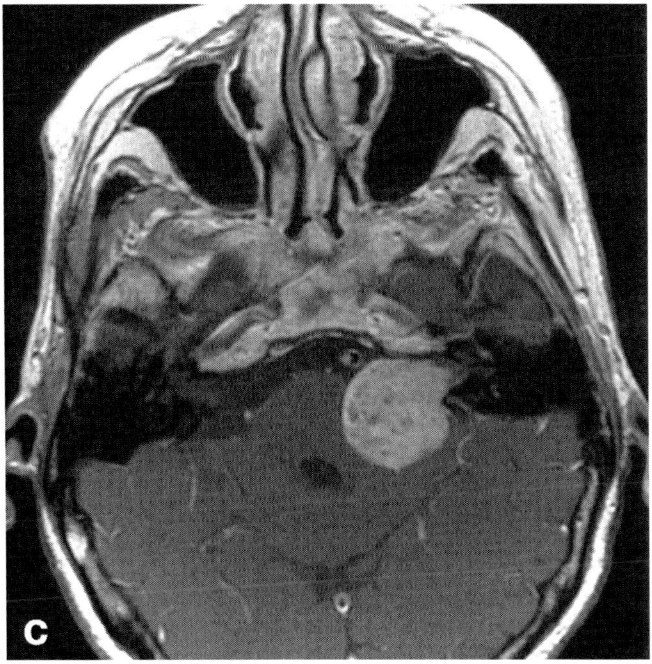

Figure 4. Giant vestibular schwannoma with typical "ice cream on cone" pattern (same patient shown in Figure 2): T2-w TSE with fat saturation (a), T1-w TSE scanned before (b) and after i.v. administration of contrast agent (c). Typical neuroradiological findings of a small intracanalicular vestibular schwannomas. The tumor arise from the internal auditory canal that is evidently widened ("the cone") and grows up by progressively occupying the cerebellopontine angle ("the ice cream") dislocating the neighboring structures of the brainsteam.

VS eroding the posterior edge of the porus acusticus it may give rise to a round component in the CPA cistern, giving the typical "ice cream on cone" pattern (Figure 4).

Small, purely intracanalicular schwannomas exist, but may also present with a dumbbell extension in the cochlea (Figure 5) or vestibule [13]. On the other hand, purely intracisternal vestibular schwannomas, without IAC involvement, have a large space to grow in before becoming symptomatic, and at imaging are always larger and heterogeneous due to cystic components (Figure 6a) or bleeding (Figure 6b) [14].

Enhancement of the adjacent meninges is possible in vestibular schwannoma and is not specific nor exclusive for meningiomas [15].

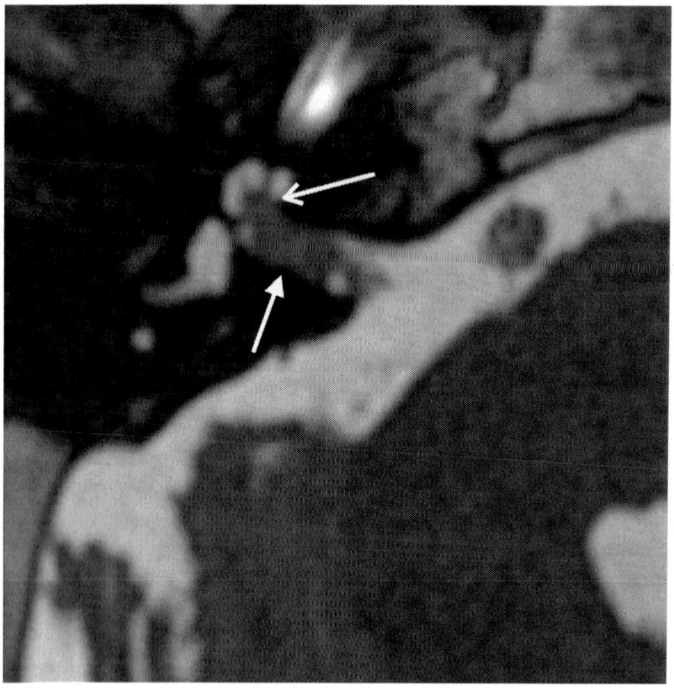

Figure 5. Right small intracanalicular schwannomas (arrow) with dumbbell extention to the cochlea (empty head arrow) appears as a hypointense mass on axial 3D CISS.

There are described three different MRI appearances of the tumor after contrast agent administration: homogeneous (50 – 60%), heterogeneous (30 – 40%), and cystic (5 – 15%) [16].

MRI may be used also to optimise treatment planning with respect to several features of the lesion:

a. the size of the tumour;
b. the distance between the lateral extremity of the intracanalicular portion of the tumour and the fundus because it affects the hearing prognosis and may modify the surgical approach;
c. the intralabyrinthine signal intensity: poor hearing prognosis may be predicted by a low T2-signal intensity of labyrinth contents compared to the unaffected ear;
d. the identification of the facial nerve and its position relative to the vestibular schwannoma [9].

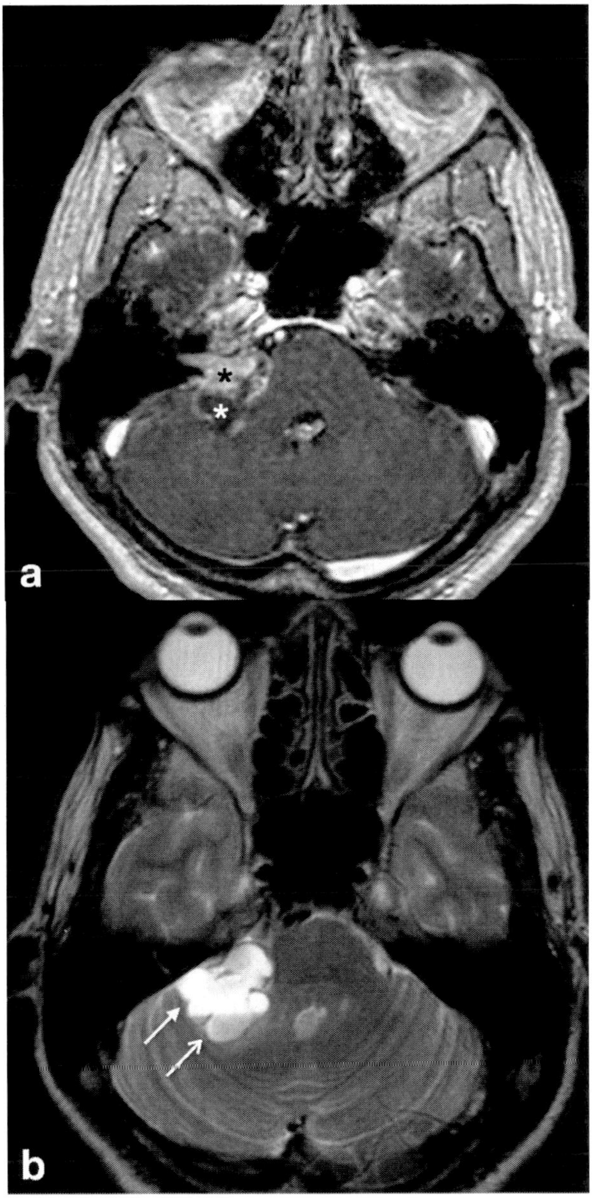

Figure 6. Heterogeneous giant vestibular schwannoma carachterized by a solid component arising from the right IAC and esxtending to the CPA cistern (black asterisk in a). The posterior-inferior part of the tumor is essentially cystic (white asterisk in a) with a fluid-fluid level to be related to recent bleeding (fluid filled cystic component in indicated by the arrow in b; the empty head arrow indicates the bleeding).

3. Differential Diagnosis

The CPA lesions that may mimic a VS include: meningioma, aneurysm, epidermoid cyst, lipochoristomas, dermoid cyst and intra-axial tumors with CPA involvement.

Meningioma represents the second most frequent (10% – 15%) tumour of the CPA after VS [8].

It is usually located at the posterior aspect of the temporal bone or at the premeatal area, from where it can easily extend into the IAC but, in opposition to VS, without enlarging the porus [9]. At CT, meningiomas are hyperdense in 70% of the cases, calcified in about 20% and show a frequent adjacent bone reaction including hyperostosis and enostotic spur.

Meningiomas are isointense to brain cortex on all pulse sequences, and strongly enhance after i.v. contrast agent injection, usually with a homogeneous pattern. The "dural tail sign", is particularly frequent in association with meningiomas, but not specific [15] and should suggest the diagnosis when observed.

An aneurysm may also mimic VS, especially on CT, because they appear as well defined round lesions that enhance after contrast administration. The vertebral and basilar arteries and some of their branches pass through the CPA cistern, where an aneurysm can develop. At MRI, aneurysms without internal thrombus have flow voids and pulsation artefacts on all spin echo pulse sequences but demonstrate iso-to-high signal intensities and variable patterns of gadolinium uptake on T1-w images when intraluminal thrombus is present. MR angiography should then be performed to confirm the diagnosis, detect the parent artery and plan the possible therapeutic options [17].

Epidermoid cyst is the third most frequent tumor of the CPA [7]. These tumours grow slowly encasing nerves and arteries in the cisterns with a specific cauliflower-like outer surface [4] without widen the IAC. On CT scans, epidermoid cysts appear hypoattenuating to CSF, and have characteristic irregular, lobulated margins. As opposed to arachnoid cyst, epidermoid cyst produces no reaction of the adjacent bone structures. At MRI, epidermoid cysts have slightly higher signal intensity than CSF on

T1w and T2w images. FLAIR and DWI sequences are well known to allow differentiation between epidermoid and arachnoid cysts. DWI offers a specific finding for epidermoid cysts by showing a very bright signal [18].

Lipochoristomas, more appropriately characterized as "lipomatous choristomas", are benign rare tumours (0.1% of all CPA tumours) that arise from mesenchyme endogenous to the vestibulocochlear nerve [19]. They typically appear as homogeneous fatty lesions surrounding and encasing normal adjacent neurovascular structures with very dense adhesions, usually asymptomatic. Sometimes they may produce symptoms by compressing the adjacent cerebral structures, such as the cranial nerves [20]. Lipochoristomas typically shows as hypoattenuating lesions on CT with a high signal on MRI T1-weighted images (promptly suppressed with fat saturation sequences) and no contrast enhancement on T1-weighted images acquired after i.v. administration of contrast medium (Figure 7).

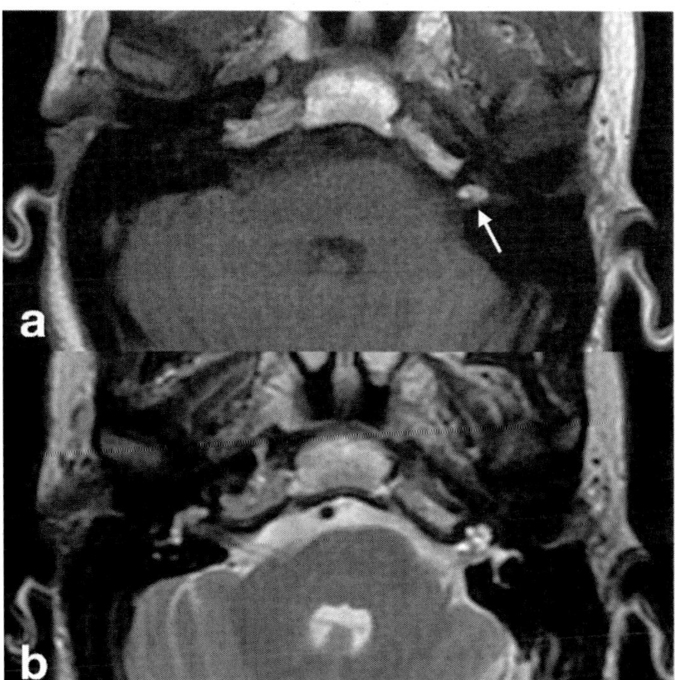

Figure 7. (Continued).

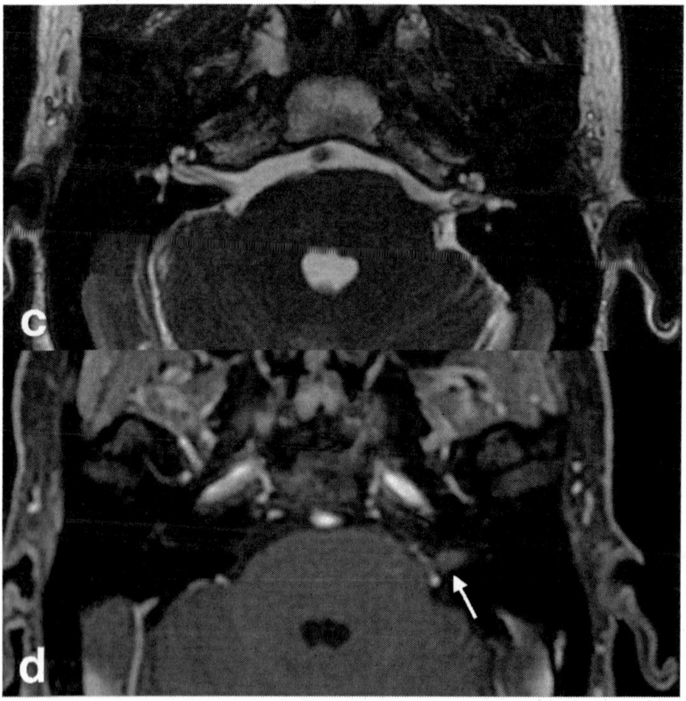

Figure 7. A small lipochoristoma occupying the left internal auditory canal. These lesions are characterized by a high signal on T1-w (a) and T2-w (b) pulse sequences, nonspecific signal on 3D CISS (c) and suppressed signal with no contrast enhancement on T1-w sequences (d).

They usually show an indolent slow growth and conservative management with periodic imaging follow-ups is thus recommended. Those lesions which has a low fat content usually show an iso- or mildly hypo-intense signal on T1-weighted pulse sequences with appreciable signs of contrast enhancement after i.v. administration of gadolinium chelate [21, 22].

Sometimes, an intra-axial or intraventricular tumor can be large enough to invade the CPA or to manifest as a CPA mass. In such a case, the intra-axial origin could be almost impossible to define. Diagnosis is difficult, but subtle signs like narrowing of the cisterns, irregularity of the tumor-brain interface, and edema are helpful. In this contest, the most frequent diagnosis includes: pedunculated brainstem glioma, choroid plexus papilloma, lymphoma, hemangioblastoma, ependymoma, medulloblastoma, dyscmbryoplastic neuroepithelial tumor (DNET) [4].

REFERENCES

[1] Juliano, A. F., Ginat, D. T., Moonis, G. Imaging review of the temporal bone: part I. Anatomy and inflammatory and neoplastic processes. *Radiology,* 2013 Oct.; 269(1):17 - 33. doi: 10.1148/ radiol.13120733.

[2] Juliano, A. F., Ginat, D. T., Moonis, G. Imaging Review of the Temporal Bone: Part II. Traumatic, Postoperative, and Noninflammatory Nonneoplastic Conditions. *Radiology,* 2015 Sep.; 276(3): 655 - 72. doi:

[3] Bonneville, F., Savatovsky, J., Chiras, J. Imaging of cerebellopontine angle lesions: an update. Part 1: enhancing extra-axial lesions. *Eur. Radiol.,* 2007 Oct.; 17(10):2472 - 82. Epub 2007 Jun. 12.

[4] Bonneville, F., Savatovsky, J., Chiras, J. Imaging of cerebellopontine angle lesions: an update. Part 2: intra-axial lesions, skull base lesions that may invade the CPA region, and non-enhancing extra-axial lesions. *Eur. Radiol.,* 2007 Nov.; 17(11):2908 - 20. Epub 2007 Jun. 14.

[5] Chavhan, G. B., Babyn, P. S., Jankharia, B. G., Cheng, H. L., Shroff, M. M. Steady-state MR imaging sequences: physics, classification, and clinical applications. *Radiographics,* 2008 Jul.-Aug.; 28(4):1147 - 60. doi: 10.1148/rg.284075031.

[6] Baráth, K., Huber, A. M., Stampfli, P., Varga, Z., Kollias, S. Neuroradiology of cholesteatomas. *AJNR Am. J. Neuroradiol.,* 2011 Feb.; 32(2):221 - 9. doi: 10.3174/ajnr.A2052. Epub 2010 Apr 1.

[7] Bonneville, F., Sarrazin, J. L., Marsot - Dupuch, K. et al. Unusual lesions of the cerebellopontine angle: a segmental approach. *Radiographics,* 2001; 21:419 - 438.

[8] Sarrazin, J. L. Infratentorial tumors. *J. Radiol.,* 2006; 87:748 - 763.

[9] Hentschel, M. A., Kunst, H. P. M., Rovers, M. M. et al. Diagnostic accuracy of high-resolution T2-weighted MRI vs. contrast-enhanced T1-weighted MRI to screen for cerebellopontine angle lesions in symptomatic patients. *Clinical Otolaryngology,* 2018; 43:805 - 811.

[10] Casselman, J. W., Kuhweide, R., Deimling, M., Ampe, W., Dehaene, J., Meeus, L. Constructive interference in steady state-3DFT MR imaging of the inner ear and cerebellopontine angle. *AJNR Am. J. Neuroradiol.,* 1993 Jan.-Feb.; 14(1):47 - 57.

[11] Giesemann, A., Hofmann, E. Some Remarks on Imaging of the Inner Ear: Options and Limitations. *Clin. Neuroradiol.,* 2015 Oct.; 25 Suppl. 2:197 - 203.

[12] Schmalbrock, P. Comparison of three-dimensional fast spin echo and gradient echo sequences for high-resolution temporal bone imaging. *J. Magn. Reson. Imaging,* 2000 Dec.; 12(6):814 - 825.

[13] Salzman, K. L., Davidson, H. C., Harnsberger, H. R. et al. Dumbbell schwannomas of the internal auditory canal. *AJNR Am. J. Neuroradiol.*, 2001; 22:1368 - 1376.

[14] Gagliardo, C., Martines, F., Bencivinni, F., La Tona, G., Lo Casto, A., Midiri, M. Intratumoral haemorrhage causing an unusual clinical presentation of a vestibular schwannoma. *Neuroradiol. J.,* 2013 Feb.; 26(1):30 - 4. Epub 2013 Mar. 8.

[15] Guermazi, A., Lafitte, F., Miaux, Y. et al. The dural tail sign-beyond meningioma. *Clin. Radiol.,* 2005; 60:171 - 188.

[16] Gomez-Brouchet, A., Delisle, M. B., Cognard, C. et al. Vestibular schwannomas: correlations between magnetic resonance imaging and histopathologic appearance. *Otol. Neurotol.,* 2001; 22:79 - 86.

[17] Papanagiotou, P., Grunwald, I. Q., Politi, M. et al. Vascular anomalies of the cerebellopontine angle. *Radiologe,* 2006; 46:216 - 223.

[18] Liu, P., Saida, Y., Yoshioka, H., Itai, Y. MR imaging of epidermoids at the cerebellopontine angle. *Magn. Reson. Med. Sci.,* 2003; 2:109 - 115.

[19] Scangas, G., Remenschneider, A., Santos, F. Lipochoristoma of the Internal Auditory Canal. *J. Neurol. Surg. Rep.*, 2015 Jul.; 76(1): e52 - e54.

[20] Sade, B., Mohr, G., Dufour, J. J. Cerebellopontine angle lipoma presenting with hemifacial spasm: case report and review of the literature. *J. Otolaryngol.*, 2005; 34:270 - 273.

[21] De Stefano, A., Kulamarva, G., Dispenza, F. Malignant paroxysmal positional vertigo. *Auris Nasus Larynx*, 2012; 39:378 - 382.

[22] Dispenza, F., Cappello, F., Kulamarva, G., De Stefano, A. (2013) The discovery of the stapes. *Acta Otorhinolaryngol. Ital.,* 33: 357 - 359.

In: Vestibular Schwannoma
Editors: Francesco Dispenza et al.
ISBN: 978-1-53617-191-4

Chapter 5

SOLITARY VESTIBULAR SCHWANNOMA: DECISION MAKING OF TREATMENTS

Francesco Dispenza[1,2], MD, PhD, Antonina Mistretta[2], MD, Barbara Verro[2], MD, Francesco Lorusso[2], MD, Ignazio La Mantia[3], MD and Alessandro De Stefano[4], MD, PhD

[1]Istituto Euromediterraneo di Scienza e Tecnologia – IEMEST, Palermo, Italy
[2]U. O. C. Otorinolaringoiatria Azienda Ospedaliera Universitaria Policlinico P. Giaccone, Palermo, Italy
[3]U. O. C. Otorinolaringoiatria Policlinico Universitario, Catania, Italy
[4]U. O. Audiologia Foniatria Ospedale V. Fazzi, Lecce, Italy

ABSTRACT

Therapeutic strategies of vestibular schwannomas treatment are changed in the last years. The improvement of surgical equipments and skills allowed increasing the *number* of successful operations in the last 10 years. The results improved in terms of survival, quality of life, recurrences, facial nerve function, and hearing preservation. Also, the age of operated patients, once a restriction, becomes progressively a relative limitation to surgical indication.

However, the progressive widening of MRI availability gives to the Otoneurologist the possibility to follow-up the patients with a *relatively* simple radiological examination, delaying the decision to treat surgically the neoplasm only in case of growth or symptoms occurrence.

The medical society is in demand of a treatment strategy based on hard data especially on the growth pattern of these tumors.

To have a complete picture of the treatment options we will discuss following the several *modalities* to manage a solitary vestibular schwannoma; the discussion about radiotherapy-radiosurgery is treated elsewhere in this book.

INTRODUCTION

Vestibular schwannomas are benign, slow growing tumors that arise from the vestibular-cochlear nerve. This neoplasm was also called: acoustic neurinoma, acoustic neuroma or more generally acoustic tumor. They arise from the Schwann cells of the nerves composing the acoustic bundle and are characterized by a slow growth, although not well estimable. The vestibular schwannoma could be part of a systemic disease called Neurofibromatosis type 2, in which the acoustic tumors are bilateral and more aggressive. Vestibular *schwannoma represents* about 6% of all intracranial tumors and accounts for about 80% of all tumors diagnosed in the cerebello-pontine angle (CPA). The incidence reported is 10-20:1000000 per year (Stangerup et al. 2006). Both *sexes* are involved equally and there is not race prevalence. The incidence increased in the last 10 years, but it was due to the enlarged availability of MRI done for others reasons. However, the true incidence could be different and greater than actually known, *because* a lot of tumors remain silent and undiagnosed.

The typical presentation of the solitary vestibular schwannoma (VS) includes: unilateral progressive sensorineural hearing loss (SNHL) in the high frequency range, unilateral tinnitus and vertigo spells or imbalance. *However abnormal clinical presentation may be characterized by sudden sensorineural hearing loss or facial weakness.* Sometime VS is completely asymptomatic and diagnosed casually. Generally, the retard of diagnosis is about 5 years.

The treatment options for patients with VS consist in: total or subtotal surgical excision, radiotherapy (Gamma Knife stereotactic radiosurgery and fractionated stereotactic radiotherapy with linear accelerator) and conservative management with serial observation by magnetic resonance imaging (MRI) scanning.

NATURAL HISTORY AND CLINICAL OVERVIEW

The large part of vestibular schwannomas is a benign slow growing tumor and the natural course of the disease is unreadable. The tumor may grow continuously or until a certain size, and then it can stop the growth for an incalculable time. Although slow, the growth rate is not estimable and the regulating factors are still unknown. It was estimated that the size of acoustic tumor increases in diameter at an average of 1 to 2 mm per year. In 30% to 70% a growth is demonstrable over a variable period of time, but in some *patients*, we can observe a spontaneous tumor regression. The variable percentage of growth reported may depend, at least in part, on the length of the observation period (Charabi et al. 2000). In a consistent number of cases the size of tumor *remains* stable for a long period and after 5 years the growth seems to be arrested. However, it is probable that most tumors, apparently stable, will eventually exhibit a progression if observed for a decade or longer. A rapid growth could be present in some tumor with cystic component due to accumulation of fluid into cystic space or to an improvise hemorrhage (Dispenza et al. 2008), such type of tumor is quite rare. *Also*, a malignant type of vestibular schwannoma could be rarely diagnosed, but is characterized by worse prognosis and different treatments. Progressive growth in the CPA will eventually lead to compression of the brainstem and/or the cerebellum, occlusion of the fourth ventricle, and subsequently its incarceration. This is the most dangerous eventuality, and the surgical removal becomes mandatory. The growth rate is not related with sex and age of patients, as noted by some Authors (Herwadker et al. 2005).

It has been proposed that VS may arise in the region of the transition zone between the central and peripheral myelin, also known as the Obersteiner-Redlich zone. Classically, histopathologic examination of VS reveals two morphologic patterns: Antoni A and B. Antoni type A describes a densely packed cells with small, spindle-shaped, densely staining nuclei. Antoni type B refers to a looser cellular aggregation of vacuolated, pleomorphic cells. The Antoni B seems to occur in particular in large tumors.

The typical manifestations of VS include: unilateral progressive *sensorineural* hearing loss (SNHL) 68.1%, unilateral tinnitus 49.1%, and disequilibrium 50%. These symptoms can occur in various associations. Several audiological features can be present in clinical practice as unilateral sudden *sensorineural* hearing loss (4-26%) and normal hearing (4-12%). Uncommon symptoms are: headaches (10.5%), otalgia, trigeminal neuralgia (9%), facial nerve palsy (6%), cerebellar dysfunction, hydrocephalus (4%) and lower cranial nerve or brainstem related symptoms. Besides some Authors described atypical presentation of VS patients with characteristic of *Ménière's* disease or benign paroxysmal positional vertigo.

The SNHL is unilateral and slowly progressive in the history of the disease. Disturbance in word recognition over the phone is one of the first symptoms that lead the patients to the physician. The hearing may be also fluctuating mimicking a Meniere's disease or a sudden sensorineural hearing loss (SSNHL). In our personal series we found some patients presenting with SSNHL treated elsewhere with steroid showing a transitory improvement of the hearing (unpublished data), for this reason we recommend a complete evaluation for VS in all patients presenting unilateral SSNHL.

Unilateral tinnitus is often present associated or not with hearing loss. A vestibular schwannoma should be suspected in presence of persistent unilateral tinnitus, especially if isolated and in young patients. The presence of tinnitus at initial presentation was a significant predictor of tumor growth and may be a marker of increased biological auditory nerve activity. The predictive value of tinnitus is increased within the range of small- to medium-sized tumors whose management is most controversial.

Vestibular symptoms could be present in patients with schwannoma of the VIII *cranial nerve*. The patients most often complain a progressive imbalance rather than true *rotational* vertigo. At some stage of the disease few patients could present vertigo spells as well as unsteadiness. Also, positional vertigo was described in patients with cerebello-pontine angle tumor (De Stefano et al. 2008).

The progressive growth of the vestibular schwannoma may explicate the slow appearance of balance *disturbance*. The destruction of unilateral peripheral vestibular function by these *slow* growing tumors is gradual and facilitates the central vestibular compensation. For these reasons, in presence of big tumors, the symptoms of peripheral deficit are quite absent because the compensation was already obtained. Usually the acoustic tumor removal doesn't produce any peripheral deficit of balance, although the bony labyrinth is completely destroyed. In case of small tumors some peripheral deficit could be detected because the system is already functioning, but is distressed by the tumor effects.

The neurotological examination of patients with vestibular schwannoma often identifies signs and symptoms of peripheral and central vestibular dysfunction. In small tumors, nystagmus can be discovered in the horizontal plane beating to the unaffected side. A vertical nystagmus *may be* a sign of brainstem compression by a large tumor. The examination of the gait could show a vestibular ataxia, with deviation toward the affected side. Dizziness is also present in case of cerebellar dysfunction due to large tumors of the CPA compressing the cerebellum. The symptoms related to cerebellar compression are difficulty in manipulating objects with hands, intention tremor and wide base gait.

Trigeminal nerve compression by large tumors is the cause of hypoesthesia of the face. The clinical examination may reveal the absence or reduction of the corneal reflex in 15% of the patients.

The facial nerve is incredibly resistant to stretch and compression by the tumor growth. Very few cases of facial weakness are encountered in the clinical practice, and usually are due to large vestibular schwannomas. Hemifacial spasms, facial weaknesses with scarce auditory symptoms are more indicative of a facial nerve tumor. However, the facial function has to be assessed in preparation of the treatment; the House-Brackmann grading scale (House et al. 1985) is used to quantify the function of the nerve, in particular it is helpful *in monitoring* the post-surgical recovery. At the time of diagnosis 98% of patients have a grade 1 facial function.

Patients with large tumor of CPA can develop papilledema and hydrocephalus (Figure 1). The examination of fundus oculi should be made as integration of neurotologic examination.

The hearing *has* to be assessed in all patients with vestibular schwannoma. Unilateral complaints and symptoms should lead promptly to routine diagnostic pure tone and speech audiometry. Further instrumental assessments of hearing function should be done in case of hearing loss not explicable by another pathological mechanism. Asymmetric hearing loss is a suspicious condition, especially if associated with tinnitus. A decrease in speech discrimination score out of proportion to the pure tone loss is accepted as index of suspicion for acoustic tumor. Such phenomenon is known as rollover sign. It is to mention that numerous cases of vestibular schwannoma have not any hearing loss, but only an aural fullness may be present. The hearing threshold determination is mandatory to plan a correct treatment; it is generally reported as average of 500, 1000, 2000 and 4000 Hz (Pure Tone Average, PTA). The definition of the hearing as serviceable is generally thought as PTA threshold better than 50 dB or speech discrimination score better than 50%, or both. However, such consideration had not a large consensus and the classification of hearing status was reviewed in 2003 (Kanzaki et al. 2003). The new classification allows noting finer the degree of hearing change after surgery and makes more realistic report of results in preservation surgery. It better considers the importance of speech discrimination in the economy of the hearing with a cut off of 10% in SDS between each class (Table 1).

Table 1. Hearing Classification in patients affected by Vestibular Schwannoma

Class	PTA (dB)	SDS (%)
A	0-20	100-80
B	21-30	79-70
C	31-40	69-60
D	41-60	59-50
E	61-80	49-40
F	81-	39-0

This classification should be adopted to report both preoperative and postoperative hearing.

PTA is obtained by averaging the frequencies: 0.5, 1, 2, 4 kHz. Hearing is classified based on either PTA or SDS, which is worse. Better SDS class than PTA designates the category one class higher.

PTA = Pure Tone Average; SDS = Speech Discrimination Score; dB = decibel.

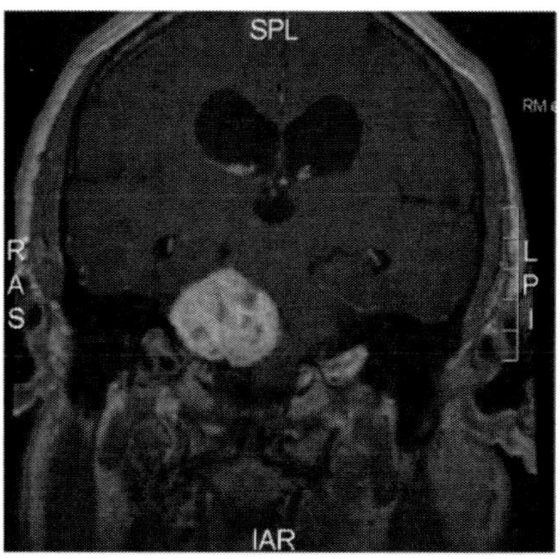

Figure 1. Giant Vestibular Schwannoma. Coronal T1 weighted MRI scan after Gadolinium enhancement shows a giant tumor of the VIII cranial nerve that displace and compress the brainstem. The only symptoms complained by this patient were: unilateral hearing loss and sight defect. It is noticeable the hydrocephalus by the enlargement of ventricles. The tumor shows solid composition with internal areas of necrosis.

The retrocochlear evaluation is still not accepted as routine examination in case of suspected acoustic tumor, and no guidelines are present about this topic. The Auditory Brainstem Responses (ABR), although advocated as useful tool to discriminate patients to undergo radiological evaluation, is not widely accepted *because it has* low specificity. The gold standard evaluation in case of suspected vestibular schwannomas remains the MRI with Gadolinium enhancement.

The MRI is the best radiological study available for diagnosis and staging of vestibular schwannoma and others CPA tumors. It allows *to visualize* the inner ear structures (i.e., cochlea and vestibule), the internal auditory canal (IAC), the CPA, and the relationship between the tumors and surrounding structures (i.e., brainstem, cerebellum, vessels, etc...). The MRI protocol includes T1-weighted images in contiguous sections through the IAC before and after contrast enhancement, and T2-weighted images obtained in section throughout the brain. On the T1 images without Gadolinium the tumor is isointense or mildly hypointense compared to the brain, after contrast enhancement the lesion appears hyperintense because of marked contrasted. On T2 images the tumor is isointense with the brain and hypointense if compared with CSF. MRI is helpful to make also some differential diagnosis preoperatively based on well-known pattern of lesions. The T2 sequences of MRI can display well the relationship between the tumor and the fundus of the IAC: the bright signal of the CSF fluid gives the size of the space between tumor and fundus (Figure 1, 2, 3, 4).

The radiological evaluation is mandatory to plan a treatment, whatever it will be and after this clinical step the size of the tumor must be evaluated. The size should be based on measurement on MRI or CT (if MRI is not feasible) of the greatest extrameatal tumor diameter (Kanzaki et al. 2003). The intrameatal portion should be clearly distinguished. If the tumor is only intrameatal (intracanalicular), without any extension out of the porus, the terms intrameatal tumor should be used (in such cases the extrameatal size is 0 mm). The intrameatal size can be measured separately in millimetres along the length of the internal auditory canal and this portion should not be added to the final size of the tumor. This measurement system was ideated to standardize the reports of the results (Table 2).

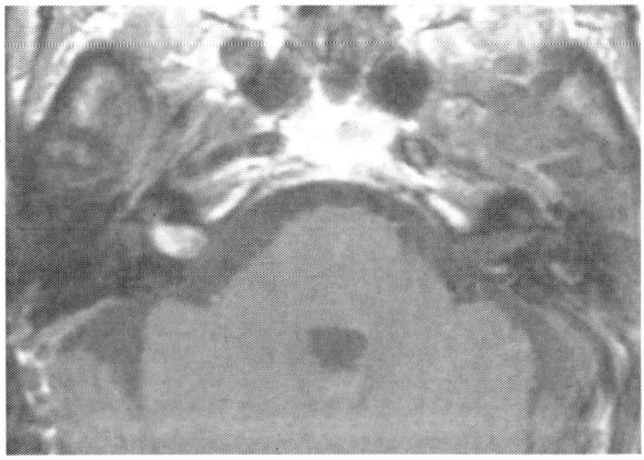

Figure 2. Intracanalicular vestibular schwannoma. Axial T1 weighted MRI scan after Gadolinium enhancement showing a tumor that is content into internal auditory canal without extrameatal component (size 0 mm). The fundus in this case is completely occupied by the tumor with an initial invasion of the cochlea. In this patient every attempt to preserve hearing with surgical approach will be disastrous.

Table 2. Tumor size classification

Grade	Description	Extrameatal Size (mm)
	Intrameatal Tumor	0
1	Small	1-10
2	Medium	11-20
3	Moderately Large	21-30
4	Large	31-40
5	Giant	> 40

The size should be based on measurement of the largest extrameatal diameter on Magnetic Resonance (Computed Tomography if MRI is not practicable). It should be noted always whether the fundus is empty or if the tumor is cystic. The size of intrameatal portion can be measured in millimeters along the length of the internal auditory canal, but this measure has not to be added on the final size. Actually is the widest accepted classification that allows to report results with quite all MRI device worldwide.

mm = millimeters.

In the clinical stage of the evaluation two characteristics of the tumor have to be noted: the state of the fundus of the internal auditory canal and the tumor morphology at MRI. The involvement of the IAC fundus is a negative predictor factor for hearing preservation surgery, as consequence it should be noted whether the fundus is empty. The nature of the tumor may be a factor that entails challenging surgical problems. Is generally considered more difficult to remove cystic tumors than solid homogeneous tumor, for this reason cystic tumors should be considered as a separated group. Cystic vestibular schwannomas (CVS) differ from solid schwannomas by their rapid growth, frequent involvement of facial nerve, and somewhat unpredictable biologic behavior. Cystic vestibular schwannomas have been estimated to represent anywhere from 5.7 to 48% of all vestibular schwannomas. A classification (Table 3) of this type of VS was recently proposed (Piccirillo et al. 2009). Factors that lead to unfavorable surgical outcomes include engulfment of and adherence to neurovascular structures, hypervascular solid portions of the tumor. Theoretically, CVS could form because of 1 or a combination of the following mechanisms: tumor growth and subsequent central necrosis, coalescence of microcysts formed in Antoni B tissue, and/or repeated intratumoral hemorrhage. Later, gradual cyst enlargement could be attributed to osmotic gradients set up by extravasation of serum proteins from an impaired blood-tumor barrier and/or the production of mucinous material within the cyst. Recently, high levels of proteolytic enzymes (matrix metalloproteinase 2) have been identified in CVS fluid and cyst walls.

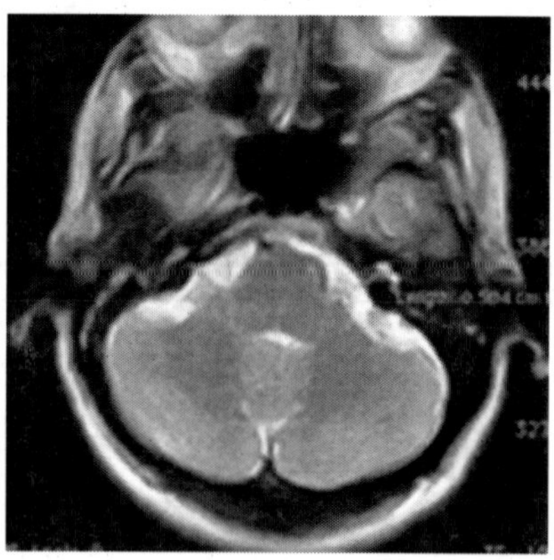

Figure 3. Intracanalicular vestibular schwannoma. Axial T2 weighted MRI scan showing a tumor confined into internal auditory canal. No extrameatal component is present. The green line shows the right orientation to measure the tumor length inside IAC.

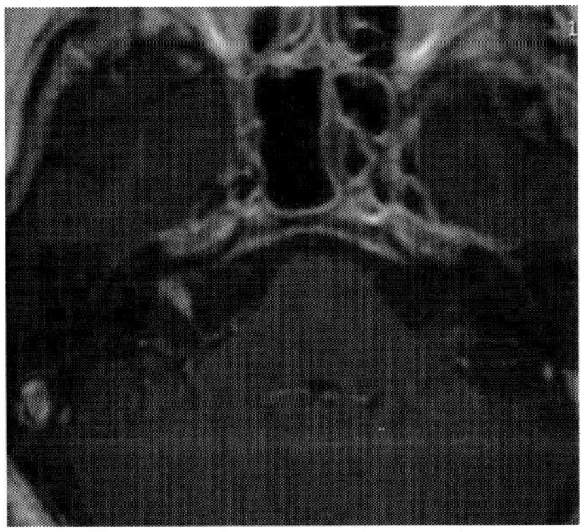

Figure 4. Cystic Vestibular Schwannoma. Axial T1 weighted MRI scan after Gadolinium showing a tumor with prevalent cystic component. The contrast enhancement is present in the minimal solid component (central portion) and in the peripheral sheath.

Table 3. Sanna's classification for cystic VS

Type	Cyst location/Wall thickness	Subtype	Definition
A	Central/thick wall	1	Polycystic (small intratumoral cysts)
		2	Polycystic (moderate size intratumoral cysts)
		3	Monocystic (single large cyst
B	Peripheral / thin wall	1	Anterior
		2	Medial
		3	Posterior
		4	Combined

The classification is based on overall cyst location (central or peripheral) and cyst wall thickness (thick or thin). Type A lesions are further subdivided by the cyst characheristics as polycystic or monocystic and its size. Type B lesions are further classified according to cyst orientation with respect to the internal auditory meatus.

CONSERVATIVE MANAGEMENT

The aim of all therapies should be to prevent morbidity and mortality in the safest, non-invasive fashion that can yield effective results. For this reason, the management of VS has shifted in recent decades away from microsurgical resection toward more conservative strategies. Vestibular schwannoma *has* all the characters of a disease manageable with the simple observation for a long period: slow growth, benign behaviour, and few symptoms in early phases. Additionally, the localization of the disease requires important surgical procedures to remove the lesion that may produce more disabling effect than the tumor itself. Furthermore, a considerable number of tumors seem to be quiescent and do not become clinically significant within a patient's lifetime; such tumor may never warrant treatment.

The conservative management consists of observation of the tumor without any active treatment, delaying the treatment until the lesion exhibits a dangerous modification.

Vestibular schwannomas are being diagnosed earlier and smaller because of improvement of imaging techniques and aggressive audiological screening in case of patients with tinnitus, dizziness, facial nerve weakness and unilateral hearing loss.

The two face of the medal are that delaying the treatment until the patient has an increase in symptoms is not likely in the patient's best interest since there is greater morbidity associated with treatment of larger tumors. On the other hand, is discussable to treat a patient with a potentially risky surgical or radiation procedure when the tumor would not have grown.

The studies done on natural history of vestibular schwannomas had several points to determine: identification of predictive factors of growth, growth rate throughout the time and the impact of observation treatment option to the health of the patients.

Conservative management of VS have been reported since 1985 (Wazen et al. 1985), these authors reported 21 elderly patients monitored with serial CT scans who undergone partial tumor removal or had not been operated on. From this beginning successive reports affirmed that the majority of VS grew during the follow-up period. Others Authors reported 50 patients who benefited from wait and see policy; 78% had growth rate of <2 mm/year (Nedzelski et al. 1992). In a big observational study of the

Danish Neurotologic school emerged that VS exhibit growth only in the first 5 years after diagnosis (Stangerup et al. 2006).

The results of our unpublished study (because of doing a long-term observational study) supported the current thought that VS are slow-growing tumors and in our series the growth was present in 42,18% of patients but the growth rate is no linear and there were not present predictive growth factors yet.

It should be noted that, although serial observation may represent the conservative management, it is not without risks. Deferring definitive treatment may lead to progression of hearing impairment or to evolution from an easily respectable lesion to one that carries increased surgical risks.

The growth of VS is not related to the final symptoms but the presence of the tumor represent for the patient in follow-up a severe risk of personal status worseness, in fact audiological deterioration can occur in the absence of evidence of tumor growth, such data leads to speculate that the sensorineural hearing loss associated with VS arises not only from the pressure effect on the internal auditory artery and/or to the cochlear nerve (Walsh et al. 2000), but perhaps also because of the deposition of tumor proteins within the inner ear (Silverstein et al. 1985).

The tumor size at initial presentation seems to be predictive of tumor growth. However the diagnosis of VS does not occur at a uniform stage in their natural history, then the tumor size at diagnosis may reflect a biological proclivity for growth, such that the detection of a large tumor at initial presentation may be indicative of past growth; to consider it as a marker for future growth potential is only a supposition.

As showed by several works, the young age is not a positive predictor of growth (Fucci et al. 1999; Herwadker et al. 2005; Stangerup et al. 2006). More aggressive treatment in younger patients based on faster tumor growth is therefore not justified by scientific observations, although other reasonable rationales for early intervention include higher cumulative lifetime risk of tumor growth and complications as well.

Conservative management presents an important concern to find the appropriate and accurate means to evaluate the tumor growth. The two main parameters to conduct a correct follow-up of the patients are: measurement of the tumor size and timing of MRI scans.

A wrong method of size measurement leads the observer to misinterpretation of the tumor behaviour and a wrong treatment may be the consequence. A two-dimensional measurement on CT, and successively on MRI, has been the method most used (Wazen et al. 1985; Nedzelski et al. 1986). In 2003 the Tokyo Consensus Meeting on System for Reporting Results in Vestibular Schwannoma accepted the measuring system, described before, with the measurement of the largest extrameatal diameter of the tumor (Kanzaki et al. 2003). Actually, is still the widest adopted system because of applicable in quite all institution with all type of MRI devices (Table 3).

Nowadays tumor size can be calculated by estimating the mean of the supero-inferior and medio-lateral tumor extent. More recently volume measurement of the tumor was proposed as an alternative to two-dimensional measurement. Interest in volume measurement comes up from the variable rate between diameter and volume in non-spherical VS, which is the most frequent manifestation. A mathematical formula based on medio-lateral and antero-posterior measures for obtain the volume of tumor was proposed (Charabi et al. 1995). A computer program can calculate volume of tumor also during the MRI scans. However, the results of tumor volume determination, obtained by mathematical formulas or computer program, were not similar especially for large VS (Shin et al. 2000). The volumetric determination of relative growth rate is becoming widely accepted because 2 mm growth in a 4 mm tumor is radically different from 2 mm growth in a 30 mm tumor, considering the rate of cellular proliferation. We advocate very strongly to counsel the patients to do MRI scans always in the same institute, avoiding differences in parameters and measurement that can alter the growth evaluation.

Another problem of conservative strategy is the non-observance of this management by the patients or *patient lost* during the follow-up. Although this non-observance has not been reported in English literature, we think that it *represents* an important difficult in this strategy. Some reasons for this non-observance may be the following: absence of traditional protocol for VS may lead patients to obtain a second opinion in other centre that applies a different policy, or patients with few symptoms may tend to wait until their hearing worseness, or elderly population with other diseases.

Today our criteria for the follow-up program are: patients with intrameatal or small – medium sized tumor (0 mm to 20 mm extrameatal) having good hearing without disabling vertigo, who refuse conservative surgical approach, patients older than 65 years, elderly patients with poor performance status, patients with only hearing ear, and patients who refuse surgery. Also in case of intralabyrinthine schwannoma, we suggest a conservative strategy in case of patients with serviceable hearing, because of whatever surgical treatment will cause anacusis in case of complete removal (Di Lella et al. 2007).

The follow-up program is developed with a yearly MRI for 5 years, followed by MRI every other year for 4 years, and a new MRI after 5 years. After such period the observation is terminated if the tumor don't show new growth or some disabling symptoms occur. This protocol can be applied generally on all VS, but some case may require a variation in MRI scheduling.

The controversy, however, continues to surround the relative merits or otherwise of conservative management with observation. The clarification of this situation is the accurate measurement of outcomes that, over the past two decades, were clinician-assessed measurement. Today the outcome measurement is shifted to a patient-assessed outcome. One of the major methods of assessing the global impact of any intervention on patients is measurement of the healthy related quality of life.

SURGICAL TREATMENTS: INDICATIONS

The modern neurotology began in early '60 when William House starts the employing of the operating microscope in his surgical approach to the neurotologic diseases. An important concept that emerged by the work of House's equip in the successive years was the multidisciplinary approach, combining the expertise of neurotologists and neurosurgeons. Such cooperation leads to the definition of the three techniques adopted by all institution worldwide: translabyrinthine, middle cranial fossa and retrosigmoid approaches to the cerebello-pontine angle.

The detailed description of the procedures is remanded to other chapters of the present book; our aim will be to address on its use in the otoneurological practice, discussing the advantage and disadvantage of the various techniques.

The translabyrinthine approach (TLA) is the most commonly used in VS removal. It allows the exposure of the CPA anterior to the sigmoid sinus, including the lateral aspect of the pons, the ventral aspect of the lateral cerebellar hemisphere and V, VI, VII, VIII cranial nerves. Also, the root entry zone of the lower cranial nerves is visible at variable angulations, depending on anatomy of the jugular bulb. The translabyrinthine approach is ideal for about all lesions of the CPA in patients without serviceable hearing and has a somewhat lower morbidity if compared to other approach that require brain retraction.

The incidence of postoperative headache is reduced because of no cerebellar retraction, completion of bony work before dura opening, scarce dissection of suboccipital musculature. The CSF leak is a rare complication following this technique. The direct and anterior prospective of view during a translabyrinthine approach allows the identification of the facial nerve at the lateral end of the internal auditory canal before the tumor dissection, and may also allow the facial nerve repair in case of accidental damage by a graft or a single anastomosis after nerve mobilization.

The main disadvantage of the translabyrinthine approach is the need to sacrifice definitively the hearing in the operated side.

The indications for this procedure generally are: nonserviceable hearing for any size of tumor, tumors larger than 2.5 cm regardless the status of the hearing. Exceptions to this rule exist in presence of particular condition (i.e., contralateral deafness).

The middle cranial fossa approach (MFA) was adopted for small acoustic tumors with good hearing. This technique allows unroofing the IAC and the exposure of its fundus. The facial nerve, located at the lateral end of the canal where it enters the temporal bone, can be visualized and dissected from the tumor. The major indication for the middle fossa approach is removal of small VS with serviceable hearing. The middle fossa approach has the main disadvantage that is a difficult approach. Because the superior location of the facial nerve in the canal, the dissection of the tumor cause more manipulation of the nerve than in other procedures with following facial nerve palsy. The retraction of the temporal lobe of the brain may become a problem in case of prolonged duration of the operation, causing seizures, memory loss, auditory hallucinations, and speech disturbances. Although rare, a bleeding in the posterior fossa could be difficult controlled because limited access. Older patients do not tolerate the middle fossa approach as well as young patients due to the delicateness of the dura and retraction of the temporal lobe. Although rare, a postoperative epidural haematoma may occur and have serious consequences if not promptly recognized.

The retrosigmoid approach (RSA) was ideated as modification of the classical suboccipital approach. In the suboccipital procedure a large bone flap is removed from the suboccipital area, with the anterior limit of the dissection being the first mastoid cell. In the retrosigmoid approach, the anterior limit of the dissection is the sigmoid sinus. Superiorly, bone is removed up to the inferior margin of the transverse sinus. The retrosigmoid approach offers a more favourable angle of view into the CPA and markedly reduced need for cerebellar retraction than the classical suboccipital technique. The retrosigmoid approach give to the surgeon a panoramic view of the posterior fossa from the tentorium to the foramen magnum. Access is provided to the cerebellar hemisphere, the lateral aspect of the pons and medulla, and from the root entry zone to the cisternal course of cranial nerves V to XI. Indications include resection of VS, meningiomas, epidermoids, cranial nerves neurectomies, vascular decompression and parenchymal lesions of the brainstem and cerebellum.

Advantages are wide access to the CPA with potential for hearing preservation. The retrosigmoid approach is capable of addressing most lesions of the CPA (Atlas et al. 1992).

Disadvantages include a higher incidence of postoperative headaches and CSF leaks (Smith et al. 1990). The rationale for the higher incidence of headache is unknown, but it is thought to be due to deterioration of posterior fossa arachnoid by bone dust dropping during intradural drilling of the posterior wall of the IAC, creating a form of chronic aseptic meningitis that is responsive to steroids. Another explication for headache is the adhesion of the posterior fossa dura to the suboccipital muscles. The higher incidence of CSF leaks is explained by the difficulty in sealing all the cells in the petrous apex, especially if it is extensively pneumatized.

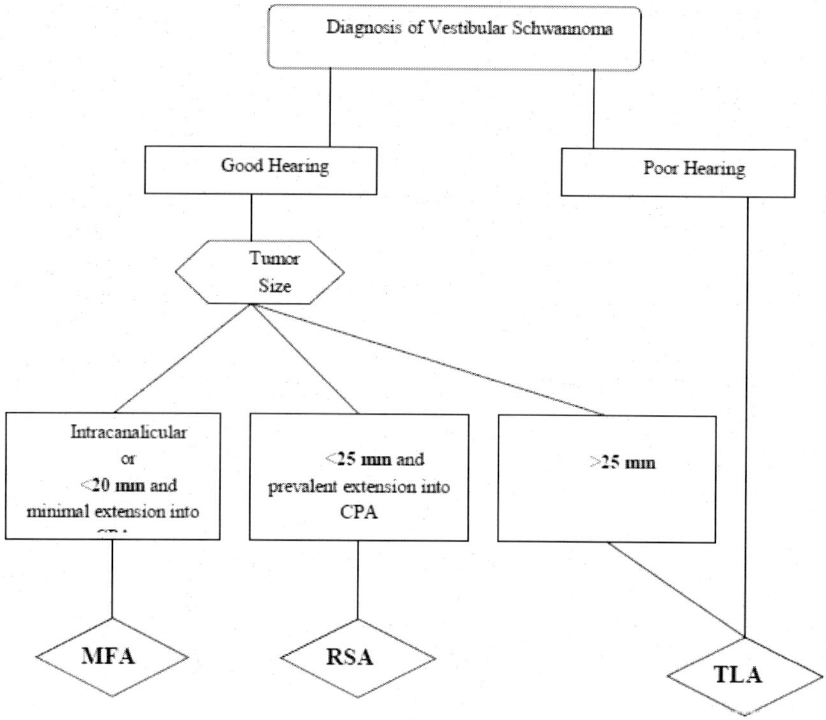

Hearing status and tumor size are the two parameters that must be considerate in choosing the proper surgical approach. Also the extension into CPA and the relationship between tumor and fundus of internal auditory canal could be restriction factors.

CPA = Cerebello-Pontine Angle; MFA = middle fossa approach; RSA = retrosigmoid approach; TLA = translabyrinthine approach.

Figure 5. Surgical management algorithm.

The aim of the surgical treatment is dual: remove a potential life-threatening disease, and preserve the hearing and facial nerve function as possible. The decision to adopt a surgical approach depends upon the characteristics of the tumor, the hearing function, the performance status of the patients and the patient's needs (Figure 5).

The concept of hearing preservation requires some explication, because often it is confused with the concept of useful hearing. Only the useful hearing is a measure of hearing preservation surgery, because it allows the patients to still benefit from hearing aids.

Several classification systems have been suggested for the description of the hearing loss. The aim of the classifications is always the standardization of communication between professionals, permitting also the comparison of treatment results.

As described before, the two most widely adopted systems are: that of the American Academy of Otolaryngology-Head and Neck Surgery (AAO-HNS) (Committee on Hearing and Equilibrium 1995), and the Gardner-Robertson system (Gardner et al. 1988). Both are based on the pure-tone threshold average (PTA) of frequencies 0.5, 1, 2, 3 kHz, as well as the best speech discrimination score (SDS). The two systems are comparable for the first two classes (A and B for AAO-HNS and 1 and 2 for the Gardner-Robertson) and this is important because many institutions consider patients for hearing preservation surgery only if their hearing falls within one of the first two classes. This behaviour is also known as "the 50/50 rule" (50 dB on PTA and 50% of SDS). A disadvantage of such systems is that the categories are too broad and a patient may drop in a worse class by loosing as little as 5 dB on one or two frequencies; this may shift the surgical option from a hearing preservation surgery to an aggressive procedure. Since 2003 a new classification system is also employed for preoperative and postoperative evaluation of useful hearing, and thus an evaluation of treatment success (Kanzaki et al. 2003). It is mandatory to stress the concept that useful hearing have to allow binaural hearing, with possible localization of sound source and discrimination in noisy backgrounds. For this, the threshold difference between the two ears should be less than 15-20 dB, with a difference of less than 15% in SDS.

Anyway, if the hearing obtained does not satisfy the above criteria, it could be suitable for amplification by hearing aids and thus contribute in binaural hearing, but only useful hearing is a measure of hearing preservation surgery. From there, the treatment should be personalized for each case by the judgment of the surgeon, based on experience and realistic chance of hearing preservation.

In the planning the proper treatment, the surgeons have to evaluate some factors: pre-operative hearing level, tumor size and location, and performance status of the patient.

A better pre-operative hearing level indicate minor compression or stretching of the VIII nerve, integrity of vascular supply to the nerve, and a hypothetic good result in hearing preservation with surgery. As showed in several studies patients with lower PTA and higher SDS scores have better possibility to preserve hearing function (Brackmann et al. 2000; Rohit et al. 2006). The audiological assessment with ABR may give further information about the chance to preserve hearing. The absence of a response is correlated with low possibility of hearing preservation (Slattery et al. 1997). The probability to preserve hearing is inversely proportional to the latency of waves I-V (Shelton et al. 1989).

The prognostic significance of tumor size was comprehensively investigated. As reported frequently, there is a significant correlation between tumor size and preserved hearing. However other institutions reported that the tumor size have not predictive significance (Brackmann et al. 2000). Effectively, the tumor size evaluation as predictive factor for hearing preservation has two main confounding factors: the method of measurement and the population selection. The selection of patients is an important bias, because the subject candidates to the hearing preservation function are already a selected subpopulation of vestibular schwannoma patients. The measurement method is still an argument of controversy, especially about the inclusion or not of the intracanalicular portion in the final size of the tumor. Generally, the size considered as limit for hearing preservation surgery is 25 mm, but in our experience a tumor more than 15 mm of size have only 10% of chance to preserve a serviceable hearing.

The intracanalicular portion of the tumor plays a role in the decision making of the surgical approach. The lateral extension into the fundus of IAC is considered a prognostic factor in terms of hearing preservation. This comes up from the anatomy of the VIII nerve, which is separate in several bundles to enter the cribriform plate of the cochlea. Tumors that completely fill the IAC have a lower rate of hearing preservation than in cases in which the fundus of the canal appears uninvolved, one to 2 mm of space between tumor and fundus has beer correlated with higher levels of hearing preservation (Colletti et al. 2005).

In patients with unserviceable hearing the translabyrinthine approach is the standard technique adopted regardless the tumor size, because this approach *gives* to the surgeon wide field for operation and low risks. The translabyrinthine approach is mandatory also for tumor larger than 25 mm not considering the hearing status, because the hearing preservation is not reasonably practicable in big sized tumor. We suggest the TLA also in those patients with tumor size more than 15 mm that choose undergo to surgical removal.

The middle fossa approach is done generally in about one third of patients. This approach is used on patients with good hearing with intracanalicular tumors, or tumor with minimal extension into CPA, generally the size should be less than 20 mm.

The retrosigmoid is done in patients with good hearing and medial tumors with prevalent extension toward CPA and minimal into IAC.

The results of the surgery are quite homogeneous, with an average of hearing preservation in about 50% of patients treated with MCF or RS; correlated with the number of treated cases, every institute may have a better *result* in one of the two techniques.

Cystic VS should have a different decisional approach, because the unpredictable growth patterns and reported cases of cyst enlargement after radiosurgery, complete or subtotal microsurgical resection is often recommended. However, literature suggests that facial nerve outcomes after cystic VS resection have been less favorable in comparison to results after removal of solid VS (Piccirillo et al. 2009). Three factors need to be considered before cystic VS resection: thickness of the cyst wall, position of the cyst, and extrameatal size of the lesion, including cystic and solid components. Vestibular schwannomas with centrally located cysts and thick cyst walls or tumors with intratumoral cystic change (both Type A) tend to be less difficult to remove. Thin-walled, Type B tumors can present a more formidable challenge. Subtotal resection is frequently warranted when tumors of this nature are encountered.

It is general idea that completely excised VS do not recur and it is reasonable to consider less than complete removal despite the attendant increased risk of regrowth. The subtotal removal may be planned preoperatively under certain conditions. A planned incomplete resection may be undertaken when a more prolonged operation is judged unwise because the patient's advanced age or performance status. Incomplete removal may be decided intraoperatively when dissection planes are poor and the surgeon think that total removal carries a high risk of damage of the facial nerve. In selected cases subtotal removal increases the odds of hearing conservation, in particular in case of contralateral ear disease. Considering the incomplete resection, it is important to distinguish whether removal has been "subtotal" or "near total" because it has substantial impact on the risk of recurrence. In subtotal excision a substantial part of tumor remains, in near total removal the residual consists of a thin capsular peel. As a general rule, the total removal of VS should be achieved whenever possible, the near total excision is most often elected when continued dissection threatens disruption of the facial nerve.

Management of Coexistent Otologic Diseases

Fortunately the existence of a Vestibular Schwannoma (VS) with a contralateral otological disease is a very rare event. However, nowadays the early diagnosis of VS caused by the advent of improved radiological imaging modalities, such as MRI, and the increased attention given to the diseases of the ear can led to the diagnosis of VS synchrony with other otological pathologies.

When this situation is present the otologist is exposed to an important management dilemma and anyone in English literature have decided a standard protocol for these patients.

The question is: which disease should be treated firstly?

Certainly a correct choice depends upon the associated disease and establishing a right protocol can be difficult. Focalizing our attention to the tumor we have three possibilities.

In the VS management the primary goal of the treatment is to ensure that there are no significant risks imposed by the VS, and then to conserve hearing and optimize the quality of life of the patient (Dispenza et al. 2008).

Non-operative management of selected patients with VS is not a new or unusual (Gardner et al. 1986). However the watchful and waiting strategy may be a correct management but, as stated before, it is not without disadvantages. The tumor may grow with consequent hearing dysfunction that may require its removal. In this case the patients lose his chance for hearing preservation surgery associated with removal of smaller VS (Naguib et al. 2005).

The risk of hearing loss is also present in the stereotactic radiosurgery as well as facial and trigeminal nerve deficit. It may block the tumor growth in the same cases but in others the tumor may continue to grow. Moreover performing the surgery after radiotherapy treatment is more demanding due the fibrosis and scar tissue.

Regarding the surgery it is obvious that the total or the partial removal of the tumor does not warrantee hearing conservation or a perfect quality of life. For these reasons no treat the tumor could be a risky choice.

All this thought become more significant if either the contralateral ear is affected by progressive hearing loss or quality of life becomes poor caused by the diseases. Then a normal protocol for the VS management could be not adequate.

In our experience we were faced with patients affected by VS and Meniere's disease and VS and contralateral otosclerosis. These pathologies are more frequent in the people and when they summarize with a VS presence can be cause of a big decisional dilemma.

Coincidence of Meniere's disease and contralateral VS represent an unusual presentation and consequently a difficult therapeutic decision-making. The main goal of treatment should be the hearing preservation and the restoration of patient normal lifestyle. It must be evaluated the true risk related to VS compared with the chances of perioperative and postoperative morbidity.

In these patients there are several problems to solve: elimination of disabling recurrent vertigo spells, management of VS and hearing preservation. In our practice we experienced 5 patients affected by this very rare condition (see the cases reported in appendix).

A Meniere's disease refractory to conventional medical treatment leads to use ablative treatments: aminoglycosides (intratympanic or systemic) or surgical procedure (endolymphatic sac decompression, vestibular neurectomy, labyrithectomy). The use of intratympanic gentamicin (IG), known since 1977 (Lange 1977), has been recommended in an attempt to minimize complications and risks involved in other procedures.

This therapeutic option was adopted by several institutions to minimize surgical risks because elderly patients and for those that refuse surgery. The total dosage of IG administrated in our patient complaint refractory MD is 81 mg (De Stefano et al. 2007).

Fluctuating hearing loss of MD usually leads to unserviceable ear in the affected side. On the other hand, VS generally have a serviceable hearing or more frequently with some degree of hearing loss. This audiological deterioration is generally related to tumoral growth and seems to be caused by pressure effect on the internal auditory artery and the cochlear nerve, but there is a significant risk of loss of serviceable hearing also in non-growing tumors. Patients with MD, even presence of moderate to profound hearing loss, and contralateral VS with serviceable hearing could be considerate having an only hearing ear (OHE) in the side of tumor (Thedinger et al. 1993).

Recent advances in surgical and diagnostic techniques for VS have markedly reduced the morbidity and mortality of patients with this type of tumor and surgical management is recommended for the majority of patients. Complications are encountered even in the hands of the most experienced surgeons. In cases of tumors smaller than 20 mm with serviceable hearing (first two class of Kanzaki Classification) the hearing preservation is achieved only in 10-30% of cases after surgical removal, this rate fell significantly in larger VS (Naguib et al. 2005). Stereotactic radiotherapy is a nonsurgical alternative in the management of VS and several studies report adequate local tumor control, but the incidence of cranial nerve injury and the risk of late complications, especially with a single large dose, remains a drawback. Hearing preservation after radiosurgical treatment was reported by several studies to be achieved in 50-70% in patients having useful hearing and unilateral tumor. This rate is not acceptable if patient present a considered OHE patient.

Based on rate of hearing preservation of non-conservative treatments as stated before and considering the small rate of tumor growth, observation result the first and the most prudent option for patients with occurrence of tumor in an OHE. Regular follow-up is made with MRI, which improved the evaluation of tumoral growth, and audiometric tests to survey the hearing function in the OHE.

During close follow-up it is possible to convert the conservative management of VS to surgical removal if there are signs of tumor growth endangering the patient's life and also if hearing in OHE deteriorate to unserviceable levels.

Because MD manifests as a peripheral auditory and vestibular disorder, those patients who develop severe to profound sensorineural hearing loss or deafness would be excellent cochlear implantation candidates (Lustig et al. 2003). Before attempt of surgical removal of the tumor in these patients we would have strongly recommended the consideration of cochlear implantation in the deaf ear affected by MD.

Our experience showed that in these rare patients affect by MD and contralateral VS, the correct management is first the treatment of MD and second a serious follow-up of the tumor. Other treatment is very dangerous for the quality of life of the patient because hearing preservation in these patients can be very difficult also using a hearing conservative surgical technique such as RS approach with simultaneous ABI positioning. For this ABI positioning should be considered a second line treatment.

The simultaneous presence of otosclerosis, a benign but disabling process with a VS a potentially life-threatening pathology is very rare.

The first description of this association was in 1973 with a detailed account of 8 patients (Clemis 1973). Except one patient described by Clemis, in which labyrinthine otosclerosis and a VS were simultaneously diagnosed, the diagnosis of otosclerosis has always antedated that of tumor. The key to tumor diagnosis in all cases presented in literature has been either the asymmetric progression of a sensorineural hearing loss (SNHL) or a sudden unilateral hearing impairment, and the differential diagnosis when such event occur should include: progressive labyrinthine otosclerosis, perilymph fistula, endolymphatic hydrops, labyrinthine vascular occlusion and cerebello-pontine angle tumor. *The presence of a disease that cause* hearing function deterioration, such as otosclerosis, may complicate the future quality of life of this patient.

We think that in these patients the future quality of life related to a sufficient hearing function is very important. For this we though that should be convenient to treat the otosclerosis firstly, because of the surgical hearing risks is only 0,18%, while the VS surgery presents a risk of hearing loss from 50 to 100% (Naguib et al. 2005).

Treating first the otosclerosis process allows us to warrant a good hearing in one ear at least. Generally, the SDS improves after stapedotomy because of thresholds are no longer at or beyond audiometric limits. Hearing aid use became easier because patients can comfortably obtain lower aided thresholds using less gain.

When otosclerosis and VS are diagnosed in the same patient the choice of the correct management is difficult and depends on some tumor factors, like tumor size, vertigo, and hearing loss. These patients have two pathologies, which lead to progressive hearing loss; consequently, is very important decide a management. In our opinion we counsel to treat only the otosclerosis process by surgery and manage with MRI and follow-up the VS.

This procedure allows recovering one hearing function and in case of failure of stapes surgery is always possible to perform a cochlear implant in otosclerotic ear (or in VS ear if the cochlea is ossified).

The coexistence of two pathologies in the same patients such as VS and MD or otosclerosis is very rare, but it represents a big problem for a correct management.

The patient *has* to properly counselled regarding variability in growth rates of VS and consequent variations of management and outcome, especially for hearing. No absolute management algorithm exists and treatment must be individualized. The main difficult in decision-making is to consider each case separately for the best therapeutic choice, keeping in mind the quality of life of the patient. Our algorithm was: treatment of disabling vertigo of MD or Hearing loss of otosclerosis and conservative management of asymptomatic VS. We recommend cochlear implantation in the deaf ear before attempt surgical removal of VS.

Vestibular schwannoma in an OHE is certainly a challenge. Because of no standard solution is available, it requires an open discussion with the patients and their relatives to choose a presumably optimal option in each case. Efforts should be made to increase the possible alternatives from which patients can select. It has been stated that the best option for hearing in such patients is to keep their own hearing and follow them with a wait-and-see policy (Naguib et al. 2005). However, the hearing preservation policy is a good option in these patients but it depends by size of the tumor, growth of it and location of the tumor (deep or lateral respect to the IAC) and rapid loss of hearing function are conditions that critically reduce chances for hearing preservation. If the tumor grow the otoneurosurgeon have some options to counsel to the patient: to remove the tumor, attempting hearing preservation; to refer the patient for radiosurgery; to remove the tumor and, if hearing is lost, to attempt cochlear implantation (provided the cochlear nerve has been spared); if possible an attempt to implant the other side should be done, and then to decide whether to remove or to follow-up the tumor; or to remove the tumor and, if the cochlear nerve is lost, to try an Auditory Brainstem Implant (ABI).

Cochlear implantation is the best method for hearing rehabilitation in patients with VS in the only hearing ear that loses hearing (Thedinger et al. 1993), certainly better than an ABI (Brackmann et al. 1993; Lenarz et al. 2001).

Cochlear implantation is usually a relatively easy procedure to perform, with no problem in identifying the correct placement of the prosthesis and negligible risk to the patient. The ABI, however, even in the most experienced hands, is not always easy and indeed may be impossible to insert. The operation does carry risk, albeit slight, to the stem and to the lower cranial nerves (Ramsden et al. 2005).

Cochlear implantation could be tried if hearing greatly deteriorates or is lost as a consequence of tumor growth or tumor removal. In the latter case, the cochlear nerve should be spared as well as the cochlea; also the vascular supply should be preserved to some degree, because otherwise the cochlea could be affected with time by fibrosis or ossification (Belal 2001). Cochlear implantation has been successful after VS removal through a retrosigmoid or a middle fossa approach. Cochlear implantation could be tried in the contralateral side, but it is advisable to remove the tumor afterwards to avoid the problem of follow up with a cochlear implant in place. The same problem is present when there are residual lesions.

Cochlear implantation after VS removal is not always possible; the cochlear nerve must be preserved intact and the cochlea should remain responsive to electrical stimulation. After removal of VS through a hearing preservation approach (i.e., retrosigmoid or middle cranial fossa) vascular supply to the cochlea may be compromised and the cochlea may ossify in the short- or mid-term (Belal 2001). If a CI is being considered, it should be performed near the time of the surgery for VS; promontory tests may help in confirming the utility of the cochlea but are not 100% reliable (Lambert et al. 1992). Basic studies have demonstrated that there could be as many spiral ganglion cells years after labyrinthectomy as in a successfully implanted patient; moreover, it has been proved that with a low population of spiral ganglion cells we can have a successful CI user (Chen et al. 1988). This supports the fact that we can use a CI after eliminating the posterior labyrinth, and in fact, placement of a CI after labyrinthectomy has proved to work properly (Facer et al. 2000).

The translabyrinthine approach for removal of VS is a highly destructive method and cochlear fibrosis or ossification occurs in a short time. If a CI is planned after such an approach, this should be done as close to the procedure as possible and optimally during the same operation. In view of histopathologic studies, it seemed reasonable that cochlear implantation could work after a translabyrinyhine approach, provided the cochlea and the cochlear nerve could be functionally preserved.

When the CI is not actable in the VS ear or in the contralateral ear the otoneurosurgeon can use an ABI implant.

The outcomes after ABI are, however, variable, and the factors that contribute to the variability are as yet not fully understood. Accurate placement of the prosthesis is essential, and this is usually possible if there has not been excessive distortion of the brain stem from a very large tumor. It is also likely that the same pressure on the stem might cause cellular depletion of the cell in the cochlear nucleus (Ramsden et al. 2005).

Several implant teams, agree that ABI confers an awareness of environmental sounds and is an adjuvant to lip-reading (Colletti et al. 2000; Lenarz et al. 2001). Nevertheless, there are reports of very good outcomes in a small proportion of patients, and the fact that this is possible at all means that there must be factors as yet largely unidentified that predict a good result. But, nowadays, the ABI is a valuable tool for cases in which the cochlea or the cochlear nerve could not be spared, for the moment, the results with ABI still are far from those obtained with CI in VS patient and OHE.

In fact before to try an ABI implant in an OHE patient we must keep in mind that tumor volume plays an important role in the alteration of the anatomic landmarks and the functional deterioration of the auditory pathways (Lenarz et al. 2001).

References

Atlas, M. D., Harvey, C. and Fagan, P. A. (1992). "Hearing preservation in acoustic neuroma surgery: a continuing study." *Laryngoscope* 102: 779-783.

Belal, A. (2001). "Is cochlear implantation possible after acoustic tumor removal?" *Otol Neurotol*\ 22\(4\): 497-500\.

Brackmann, D. E., Hitselberger, W. E., Nelson, R. A., Moore, J., Waring, M. D., Portillo, F., Shannon, R. V. and Telischi, F. F. (1993). "Auditory brainstem implant: I. Issues in surgical implantation." *Otolaryngol Head Neck Surg*\ 108\(6\): 624-33\.

Brackmann, D. E., Owens, R. M., Friedman, R. A., Hitselberger, W. E., De la Cruz, A., House, J. W., Nelson, R. A., Luxford, W. M., Slattery III, W. H. and Fayad, J. N. (2000). "Prognostic Factors for Hearing Preservation in Vestibular Schwannoma Surgery." *Am J Otol* 21: 417-424.

Charabi, S., Thomsen, J., Mantoni, M., Charabi, B., Jorgensen, B., Borgesen, S. E., Gyldensted, C. and Tos, M. (1995). "Acoustic neuroma (vestibular schwannoma): growth and surgical and nonsurgical consequences of the wait-and-see policy." *Otolaryngol Head Neck Surg* 113(1): 5-14.

Charabi, S., Tos, M., Thomsen, J., Charabi, B. and Mantoni, M. (2000). "Vestibular schwannoma growth: the continuing controversy." *Laryngoscope* 110(10 Pt 1): 1720-5.

Chen, D. A., Linthicum, F. H., Jr. and Rizer, F. M. (1988). "Cochlear histopathology in the labyrinthectomized ear: implications for cochlear \ implantation." *Laryngoscope*\ 98\(11\): 1170-2\.

Clemis, J. D. (1973). "The coexistence of acoustic neuroma and otosclerosis." *Laryngoscope* 83: 1953-1985.

Colletti, V. and Fiorino, F. (2005). "Is the middle fossa approach the treatment of choice for intracanalicular vestibular schwannoma?" *Otolaryngol Head Neck Surg* 132: 459-466.

Colletti, V., Fiorino, F. G., Carner, M., Giarbini, N., Sacchetto, L. and Cumer, G. (2000). "The retrosigmoid approach for auditory brainstem implantation." *Am J Otol* 21: 826-836.

Committee on Hearing and Equilibrium (1995). "Guidelines for the evaluation of hearing preservation in acoustic neuroma (vestibular schwannoma). American Academy of Otolaryngology-Head Neck Surgery Foundation, INC." *Otolaryngol Head Neck Surg* 113: 179-180.

De Stefano, A., Dispenza, F., De Donato, G., Caruso, A., Taibah, A. and Sanna, M. (2007). "Intratympanic gentamicin: a 1-day protocol treatment for unilateral Meniere's disease." *Am J Otolaryngol* 28(5): 289-93.

De Stefano, A., Dispenza, F., Di Trapani, G. and Kulamarva, G. (2008). "Meningioma of the cerebello-pontine angle mimicking benign paroxysmal positional vertigo." *J Otolaryngol* 37: 46-48.

Di Lella, F., Dispenza, F., De Stefano, A., Falcioni, M. and Sanna, M. (2007). "Management of intralabyrinthine schwannomas." *Auris Nasus Larynx* 34(4): 459-463.

Dispenza, F. and De Stefano, A. (2008). "Imaging of Vestibular Schwannoma with prevalent cystic component: Cystic Vestibular Schwannoma." *Otol Neurotol* 30: 681-682.

Dispenza, F., De Stefano, A., Flanagan, S., Romano, G. and Sanna, M. (2008). "Decision Making for Solitary Vestibular Schwannoma and Contralateral Meniere's Disease." *Audiol Neurootol* 13(1): 53-57.

Facer, G. W., Facer, M. L., Fowler, C. M., Brey, R. H. and Peterson, A. M. (2000). "Cochlear implantation after labyrinthectomy." *Am J Otol*\ 21\(3\): 336-40\.

Fucci, M. J., Buchman, C. A., Brackmann, D. E. and Berliner, K. I. (1999). "Acoustic tumor growth: implications for treatment choices." *Am J Otol* 20: 495-499.

Gardner, G., Moretz, W. H., Jr., Robertson, J. H., Clark, C. and Shea, J. J., Jr. (1986). "Nonsurgical management of small and intracanalicular acoustic tumors." *Otolaryngol Head Neck Surg* 94(3): 328-33.

Gardner, G. and Robertson, J. H. (1988). "Hearing preservation in unilateral acoustic euroma sucrgery." *Ann Otol Rhinol Laryngol* 97: 55-66.

Herwadker, A., Vokurka, E. A., Evans, D. G., Ramsden, R. and Jackson, A. (2005). "Size and growth rate of sporadic vestibular schwannoma: Predictive value of information available at presentation." *Otol Neurotol* 26: 86-92.

House, J. W. and Brackmann, D. E. (1985). "Facial nerve grading system." *Otolaryngol Head Neck Surg* 93: 146-147.

Kanzaki, J., Tos, M., Sanna, M., Moffat, D. A., Monsell, E. M. and Berliner, K. I. (2003). "New and modified reporting systems from the consensus meeting on systems for reporting results in vestibular schwannoma." *Otol Neurotol* 24(4): 642-8; discussion 648-9.

Lambert, P. R., Ruth, R. A. and Thomas, J. F. (1992). "Promontory electrical stimulation in postoperative acoustic tumor patients." *Laryngoscope*\ 102\(7\): 814-9\.

Lange, G. (1977). "Die intratympanale Behandlung des Morbus Meniere mit ototoxischen antibiotika." *Z Laryngol* 56: 409-414.

Lenarz, T., Moshrefi, M., Matthies, C., Frohne, C., Lesinski-Schiedat, A., Illg, A., Rost, U., Battmer, R. D. and Samii, M. (2001). "Auditory brainstem implant: part I. Auditory performance and its evolution over\ time." *Otol Neurotol*\ 22\(6\): 823-33\.

Lustig, L. R., Yeagle, J., Niparko, J. K. and Minor, L. B. (2003). "Cochlear Implantation in Patients with Bilateral Meniere's Syndrome." *Otol Neurotol* 24: 397-403.

Naguib, M. B., Cokkeser, Y. and Sanna, M. (2005). "Management of acoustic neuroma in the only hearing ear." *Eur Arch Otorhinolaryngol* 262: 127-130.

Nedzelski, J. M., Canter, R. J., Kassel, E. E., Rowed, D. W. and Tator, C. H. (1986). "Is no treatment good treatment in the management of acoustic neuromas in the elderly?" *Laryngoscope* 96(8): 825-9.

Nedzelski, J. M., Schessel, D. A., Pfleiderer, A., Kassel, E. E. and Rowed, D. W. (1992). "Conservative management of acoustic neuromas." *Otolaryngol Clin North Am* 25(3): 691-705.

Piccirillo, E., Wiet, M. R., Flanagan, S., Dispenza, F., Giannuzzi, A., Mancini, F. and Sanna, M. (2009). "Cystic Vestibular Schwannoma: Classification, Management and Facial Nerve Outcomes." *Otol Neurotol* 30: 826-834.

Ramsden, R., Khwaja, S., Green, K., O'Driscoll, M. and Mawman, D. (2005). "Vestibular Schwannoma in the Only Hearing Ear: Cochlear Implant or Auditory Brainstem Implant?" *Otol Neurotol* 26: 261-264.

Rohit, Piccirillo, E., Jain, Y., Augurio, A. and Sanna, M. (2006). "Preoperative predictive factors for hearing preservation in vestibular schwannoma surgery." *Ann Otol Rhinol Laryngol* 115(1): 41-6.

Shelton, C., Brackmann, D., House, W. F. and Hitselberger, W. E. (1989). "Middle fossa acoustic tumor surgery: results in 106 cases." *Laryngoscope* 99: 405-408.

Shin, Y. J., Fraysse, B., Cognard, C., Gafsi, I., Charlet, J. P., Berges, C., Deguine, O. and Tremoulet, M. (2000). "Effectiveness of conservative management of acoustic neuromas." *Am J Otol* 21(6): 857-62.

Silverstein, H., McDaniel, A., Norrell, H. and Wazen, J. (1985). "Conservative management of acoustic neuroma in the elderly patient." *Laryngoscope* 95(7 Pt 1): 766-70.

Slattery, W. H., Brackmann, D. and Hitselberger, W. E. (1997). "Middle fossa approach for hearing preservation with acoustic neuroma." *Am J Otol* 18: 596-601.

Smith, P. G., Leonetti, J. P. and Grubb, R. L. (1990). "Management of cerebrospinal fluid otorhinorrhea complicating the retrosigmoid approach to the cerebellopontine angle." *Am J Otol* 11: 178-180.

Stangerup, S. E., Caye-Thomasen, P., Tos, M. and Thomsen, J. (2006). "The Natural History of Vestibular Schwannoma." *Otol Neurotol* 27: 547-552.

Thedinger, B. A., Cueva, R. A. and Glasscock, M. E., 3rd (1993). "Treatment of an acoustic neuroma in an only-hearing ear: case reports and considerations for the future." *Laryngoscope* 103: 976-980.

Walsh, R. M., Bath, A. P., Bance, M. L., Keller, A. and Rutka, J. A. (2000). "Consequences to hearing during the conservative management of vestibular schwannomas." *Laryngoscope* 110(2 Pt 1): 250-5.

Wazen, J., Silverstein, H., Norrell, H. and Besse, B. (1985). "Preoperative and postoperative growth rates in acoustic neuromas documented with CT scanning." *Otolaryngol Head Neck Surg* 93(2): 151-5.

In: Vestibular Schwannoma
Editors: Francesco Dispenza et al.
ISBN: 978-1-53617-191-4

Chapter 6

Conservative Management of Vestibular Schwannoma

Elisabetta Zanoletti, Diego Cazzador and Antonio Mazzoni
[1]Unit of Otolaryngology, Department of Neurosciences,
University of Padova, Padova, Italy

Abstract

Conservative management means a low-morbidity control of disease with long term preservation of function and no post-treatment sequelae. It relates, daresay only, to small-size vestibular schwannoma. The "small size" tumor is defined as a less or equal to 10mm lesion in the cerebello-pontine angle, the Koos classification being not representative and rarely used in the otological community. The more the size increases, the less the conservative management can be successful. A balance between different conditions at diagnosis and between the pros and contra of each option has to be considered. The conservative treatment of a small tumor relates today to the possibility of hearing preservation, the choice to treat or not treat the tumor cannot leave this out of consideration. The conservative treatment means also low morbidity treatment, and there should be a better definition of what today morbidity for a small tumor is.

INTRODUCTION

Early imaging often allows *early* diagnosis of vestibular schwannoma, which gives rise to the question of: "how can this influence the prognosis?". In other words, how an early diagnosis can reduce the neurologic losses related to the therapy, or the absence of therapy, of vestibular schwannoma? Conservative management means a low-morbidity control of disease with long term preservation of function and no post-treatment sequelae. It relates, daresay only, to small-size vestibular schwannoma. The "small size" tumor is defined as a less or equal to 10mm lesion in the cerebello-pontine angle, the Koos classification being not representative and rarely used in the otological community. The more the size increases, the less the conservative management can be successful. Small vestibular schwannomas may involve normal hearing, which is defined by class A of the American Academy of Otolaryngology-Head and Neck Surgery or class A-B of the Tokyo classification [1, 2], i.e., 30 dB pure tone average (PTA) and 70% speech discrimination score (SDS). It is essential to ask *why* and *when* a small vestibular schwannoma should be treated. The importance of preventing and/or rehabilitating unilateral deafness is motivated by the fact that it is associated with a severe loss of quality of life, especially in adults, because of a consequently impaired speech recognition in noise, lack of directionality of sound and daily fatigue, with worsening with age. Preservation of hearing is thus considered the benchmark of therapy of small vestibular schwannomas: any active treatment is to offer better long-term functional results on hearing, since the results on the facial nerve are similar in the three options (observation, radiotherapy- or radiosurgery- and microsurgery). A hearing-focused approach involves the choice of the most promising options balancing the conditions at diagnosis. We propose a protocol for small vestibular schwannomas treatment (table 1), with the aim to be as much conservative as possible, balancing hearing conditions, tumor growth, patient's will, comorbidities and institutional experience at diagnosis. This involves that every, although small, tumor should be addressed for decision-making to an experienced center, where all the options are feasible.

Table 1. Protocol for small vestibular schwannomas treatment

T size mm in CPA	Decision factors	Treatment
T< 10	Good hearing (<30 db PTA/ >70% SDS)	Hearing preservation surgery (Retrosigmoid) or Observation
	Idem + risk	Observation
	Bad hearing	Observation or surgery (Tlab) + hearing rehab.
T 10-15	No growth	Observation or surgery (Tlab or Retrosigmoid)
	Growth	Surgery (Tlab or Retrosigmoid)
	Idem + risk	Radiotherapy
T 15-25		Surgery (Tlab) or Radiotherapy
T > 25		Surgery (Tlab)
	Risk	Partial Surgery (Tlab) + Radiotherapy
Any Size	Cystic tumor	Surgery (Tlab or Retrosigmoid)

CPA: cerebello-pontine angle; Tlab: translabyrinthine approach

Small Tumor and Poor Hearing at Diagnosis

When a small tumor with poor or no hearing is diagnosed, the conservative management means no further morbidity. This involves observation with sequential clinical and radiological evaluations to assess any change on patients' status and tumor characteristics. When an extrameatal growth is detected, then an active treatment should be advised in accordance with the patient [3]. When surgery is advocated, the aim is to avoid further morbidity on the facial nerve since the smaller a growing tumor is resected, the better the facial nerve outcome is [4].

When poor or no hearing are present, surgery should involve *limited* translabyrinthine approach, namely a further extension of a traditional mastoidectomy to the internal auditory canal through a drilling of the semicircular canals as to expose the vestibule, and the fundus. The space for microsurgical maneuvers allowed by the extradural approach guarantees safe exposure of the facial nerve and optimal control of the disease. The facial nerve is positively identified in two points: at the fundus, and at its root. The cerebellum is never retracted, the cerebello-pontine angle visualized and, if required, gently and safely entered and the control of the disease, as well as the facial nerve, are ideal.

The bony cavity of the mastoidectomy and "limited" translabyrinthine approach is filled with abdominal fat. A thick and fibrous layer of muscles and subperiosteal tissues, previously transected with a clear-cut incision, is sutured to keep all the obliteration firmly is site.

The drawback of this approach is post-surgical deafness: this is why it is performed only when preoperative hearing is poor, or in case of deafness, when growth is assessed. Hearing rehabilitation is feasible with this approach, a cochlear implant may be implanted into an intact cochlea if a good cochlear nerve is preserved.

In some cases of small tumors, the "limited" translabyrinthine approach is replaced today by a transcanal-transpromontorial approach to the internal auditory canal and the cerebello-pontine angle [5]. This approach avoids in principle the retroauricular scar and the filling of the bony cavity with fat. It involves the transpromontorial drilling of the cochlea. The control of the facial nerve starts at the fundus but does not combine preliminarily with the positive identification of its root. When the cerebello-pontine angle is to be entered, a further space is obtained variably adding a retroauricular incision, a canaloplasty, a drilling of the anterior wall of the canal, as well as the exposure of the internal carotid artery and the jugular bulb. The cavity is filled with fat and the external auditory canal closed, following the principle of a subtotal petrosectomy [6]. The transcanal-transpromontorial approach to the internal auditory canal, when enlarged to the critical structures and associated to the closure of the external auditory canal, may be defined also as a "transcanal-transpromontorial-prefacial-petrosectomy". Its main drawback, as well as the need of deep enlargement of the approach to critical structures and little space of maneuvers due to the diameter of the external auditory canal (although enlarged by a canaloplasty, disregarding the one-hand technique as allowed by the endoscope, of two-hands microsurgical technique as with the microscope), is that in the transpromonotial approach the cochlea is drilled to gain access to the internal auditory canal and cerebello-pontine angle, in principle preventing the positioning of a cochlear implant.

At our Institution we perform this approach, which is defined according to Fisch *endoaural*, only in cases of tumors involving primarily the cochlea, when the middle ear and the external auditory canal are fully preserved. If the approach involves a deep enlargement with a *transcanal-transpromontorial-prefacial petrosectomy* as to allow adequate exposure of the internal auditory canal, as well as the cerebello-pontine angle, we prefer a retroauricular approach with a *limited* translabyrinthine approach.

The conservative management of a small growing tumor may also involve radiotherapy (we prefer to call it radiotherapy instead of the misleading definition of "radiosurgery", because no surgery at all is performed while performing the "Cyber-" or "Gammaknife" technique). Indications are given according to the patient's age and willing, comorbidities, and the state of hearing at diagnosis. Radiotherapy offers a good control of the disease at long term (70% on a growing tumor) [7, 8] and a short-medium term favorable rates of hearing preservation when a good hearing (Class A Tokyo or A-B AAO-HNS) is present at the diagnosis, while the long-term (ten years follow-up) results are disappointing.

If hearing is poor, as it is the condition that we are dealing with, radiotherapy may be performed also when the tumor is bigger, observation is not necessarily to be interrupted at the critical size of 1.3 - 1.5 cm in the CPA as it is advisable [3, 9] if surgery follows observation. The results on the facial nerve are not so influenced by the size of tumor as it obviously is with surgery.

Small Tumor and Good Hearing at the Diagnosis

Good hearing at diagnosis is defined as a less than 30 dB PTA + more than 70% SDS together with measurable ABR, or presence at least of wave V. Although currently performed, it is evident today that the methods of investigating hearing are not adequate since they are not representative of the everyday conditions. Normal hearing at diagnosis is far from being infrequent and it relates to the most debatable issues about the small vestibular schwannoma. The choice of a multioptional therapy [9, 10], which balances each choice with its pros and contra, is the answer to a hearing-focused approach. The hearing-focused approach is the aim of the treatment, or of no-treatment, of small vestibular schwannoma with good hearing at the diagnosis since the three therapies, observation, radiotherapy and surgery differently endanger the chance of hearing preservation. A recent report [11] tried to set some evidences on hearing with long-term outcomes comparing the three options of treatment. No more than level 3 of evidence was achieved and only provisional conclusions could be stated.

OBSERVATION

Observation, or abstention from any active therapy, is considered to offer the best chances of long-term hearing preservation. Its value relies on the fact that the majority of small intracanalicular tumors does not grow or stops growing. This wait-and-see policy involves the issue that an inexorable decline of hearing occurs over time, despite no-growth.

As emerged in a representative paper [12], observation for intrameatal tumors is associated with a progressive hearing decline over the years, with a long-term good hearing (Class A according to the AAO-HNS) preservation rate of 17% and 34% of class B at 10 years. In the most favorable conditions (intrameatal tumors and SDS = 100%), hearing was maintained in 73% of the patients at 10 years follow-up, with an SDS > 70%, but with a PTA of 46 dB. According to the AAO-HNS classification, this result coincides with class B, which means a serviceable hearing and cannot be considered an excellent result. "The spontaneous arrest in the tumor's growth and the long-term hearing preservation enabled by observation alone makes it the benchmark with which every other therapy should be compared" [12]. Observation is the choice unless other treatments show better long-term results on hearing function.

RADIOTHERAPY

There is a great amount of papers claiming outstanding results on hearing preservation rates, and some authors [13] also argue that radiotherapy should be administered disregarding growth, when hearing preservation is the goal with a *proactive* function. Long-term results are rarely reported, and provisional actuarial data are often misleading [14]. The 1-, 3-, 5, 7- and 10-years rates of hearing preservation are reported at 80%, 55%, 48%, 38% and 23%, respectively in one the few papers presenting long-term results [11].

Other studies have different and better results, but at long-term the decline of hearing seems inexorable and not different compared to observation.

At our Institution, we do not send patients for primary *proactive* radiotherapy with the aim of hearing preservation but only after growth assessment [9]. Our position is that radiotherapy, should be administered only after tumor growth is confirmed [8].

SURGERY

Is deafness the natural consequence of surgery in small vestibular schwannomas? It depends, as already underlined, from the conditions of hearing at diagnosis and the choice of the surgical approach. In principle, when surgery is performed to cure a growing tumor or to attempt hearing preservation disregarding growth, a retrosigmoid approach is performed with the addition of a retrolabyrinthine meatotomy [15]. Surgical experience needs to be combined with some technical refinements concerning patients' positioning, preoperative definition of surgical landmarks on the labyrinth and the vestibular aqueduct, exposure of the posterior face of the petrous bone, and drilling of the internal auditory canal as to expose the fundus and allow space to microsurgical resection with the interface tumor-nerve under constant view. Hearing is always under monitoring in the intraoperative phase, with the ABR and, much more reliable although not easy to register, with the CNAP (cochlear nerve compound action potential).

Complications in the posterior fossa are minimized (< 0.5%) by the absence of cerebellar retraction (spontaneous retraction is obtained by the park-bench positioning and neuro-anesthesia) and gentle handling of the structures, with an adequate exposure through an appropriate craniotomy. The additional use of the endoscope helps to visualize nerves and vessels from a different perspective.

The retrosigmoid approach with the retrolabirinthine meatotomy is considered so far at our Institution the best approach to allow good results on hearing preservation surgery [9]. It is technical demanding and, as well as being decided according to the patient's willing, must combine a good, accurate preoperative selection of patients together with an experienced oto-neurosurgical setting.

As often stated, the preoperative conditions of hearing at the diagnosis influences greatly the prognosis on hearing [16]. This is evidenced in table 1 where our Institutional guidelines are exposed.

Medium Sized Tumor

If it is easy to assess what a small tumor is (we set the maximum size at 1 cm in the CPA), a medium size tumor is more difficult to define.

The critical size of 1.5 cm, which represents the cut-off point after which it is advised to stop observation [3], is set over the fact that the bigger the tumor is, the higher the possibility of facial nerve damage with surgery [4, 17]. Hearing too is difficult to preserve when the tumor is bigger than 1.5 cm. what happens between 1.0 and 1.5 cm? When judging a growing tumor, to assess if and when treatment should be proposed, there is a radiological aspect which influences the choice to shift to active treatment. In high resolution T2 MRI sequences, an important role it is played by the film of fluid which is still present or not around the extrameatal tumor. This helps in principle to give indication to the prompt surgical resection or it enables some mm of further growth during observation. When a conservative management is undertaken with observation, the wait and scan strategy should not impact negatively on the morbidity of the whole course of the treatment, when surgery is the choice. In other words, a growing tumor, unless the planned treatment is radiotherapy for which 1.5 or 2 cm size does not make the difference, the smaller the tumor is resected, the lowest the morbidity that surgery involves.

In conclusion, the conservative management of a vestibular schwannoma is:

1) A balance between different conditions at the diagnosis and between the pros and contra of each option. It is feasible and successful for facial and hearing preservation in small tumors. When growth is assessed, the choice of not-treating the tumor exposes the patient to higher risks of function deterioration, especially in surgery.
2) The conservative treatment of a small tumor relates today to the possibility of hearing preservation, the choice to treat or not treat the tumor cannot leave this out of consideration. Hearing preservation in principle must precede the further possibility of hearing rehabilitation, as natural hearing preservation should be the aim before hearing rehabilitation with cochlear implant. Moreover, the choice of the surgical approach, should not impact on the possibility of successfully positioning a cochlear implant.
3) The conservative treatment means also low morbidity treatment, and there should be a better definition of what today morbidity for

a small tumor is. Is it the possibility of avoiding surgery? Reducing scars? Reducing complications? Preservation of function? Provided that facial nerve preservation and control of disease is equally offered, in experienced centers, by the three options, hearing preservation, followed by eventual hearing rehabilitation, makes the difference. The low morbidity treatment should relate also to the *long-term* low morbidity, which means to take into consideration all the aspects influencing the choice of a therapy or of no-therapy, its whole long-course.

There follow some surgical pictures to explain the retrosigmoid approach with retrolabirinthine meatotomy and the translabyrinthine approach.

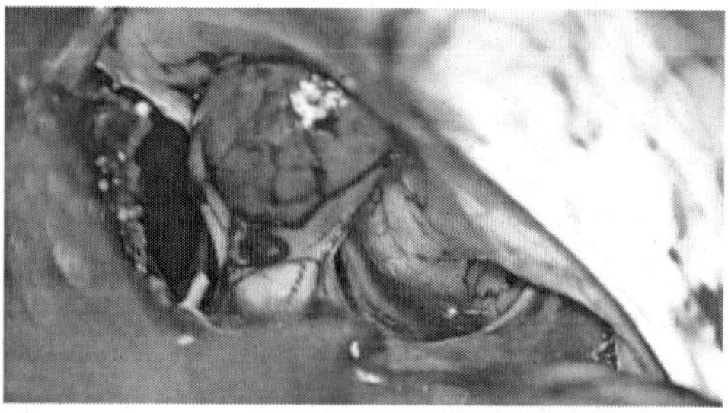

Figure 1. A small right extrameatal tumor exposed by a retrosigmoid approach. The posterior face of the petrous bone is evident, the extrameatal tumor and the root of the eight cranial nerve.

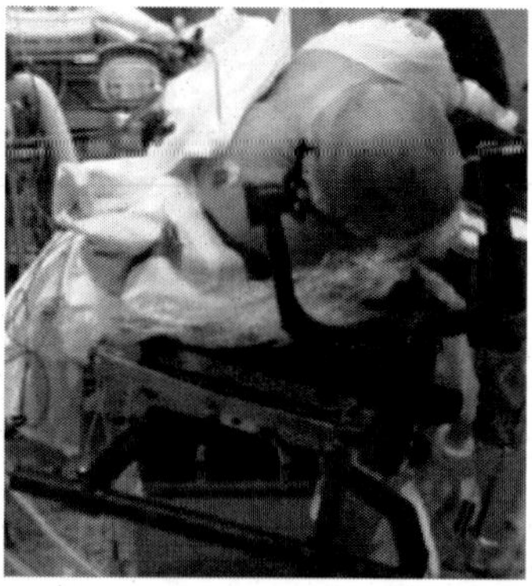

Figure 2. Park-bench positioning with an extra rotation of the surgical bed of 30°, as required intraoperatively while exposing the fundus of the internal auditory canal.

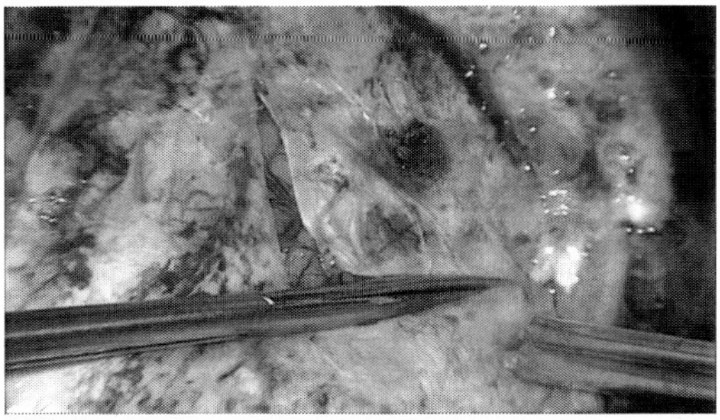

Figure 3. Right retrosigmoid approach: The craniotomy has been performed, the sigmoid and transverse sinuses are fully exposed, and the dura mater is transected in two flaps, then retracted.

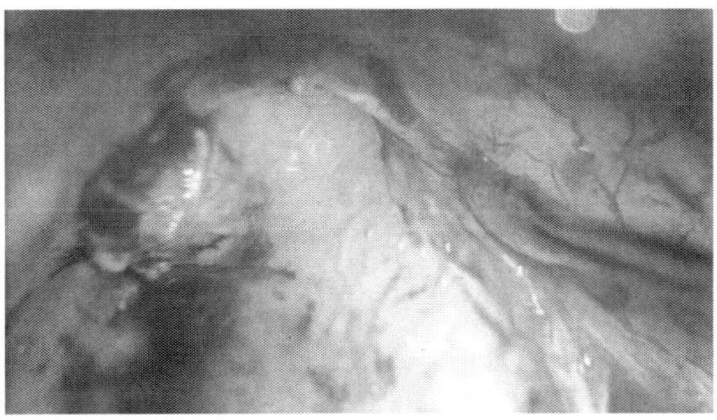

Figure 4. The posterior face of the petrous bone is exposed after transecting the dura mater covering it. The entrance of the endolymphatic sac is exposed and the ideal pathway of the vestibular acqueduct is ideally traced.

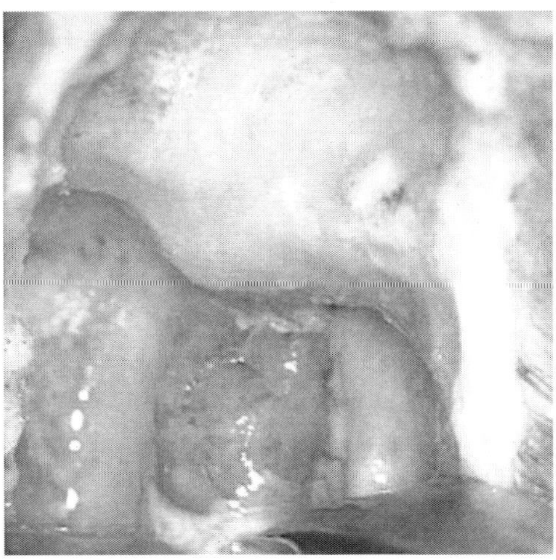

Figure 5. The surgical landmarks of the posterior and superior semicircular canals are exposed, and the blue line identified. This is the end of the retrolabyrinthine meatotomy. The intrameatal tumor is exposed.

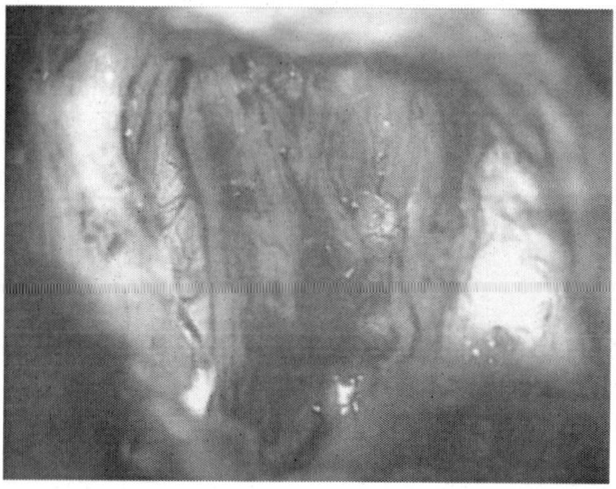

Figure 6. At the end of surgery, the facial and cochlear nerves are preserved after tumor resection.

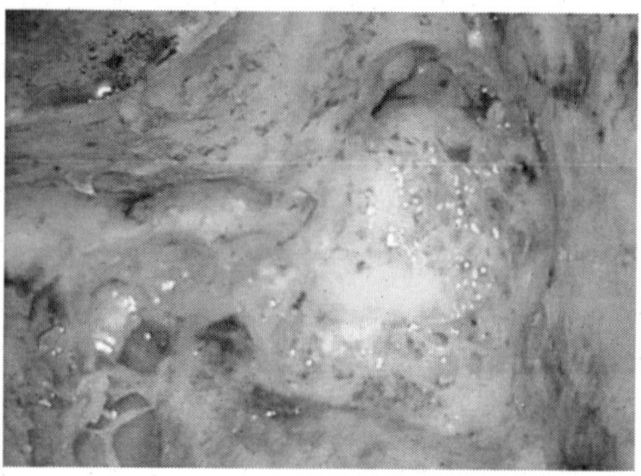

Figure 7. Left translabyrinthine approach: the labyrinth is evident with the lateral semicircular canal, the facial nerve identified in its mastoid tract, the sigmoid sinus and temporal dura mater exposed. The posterior wall of the external auditory canal and the incus are also evident.

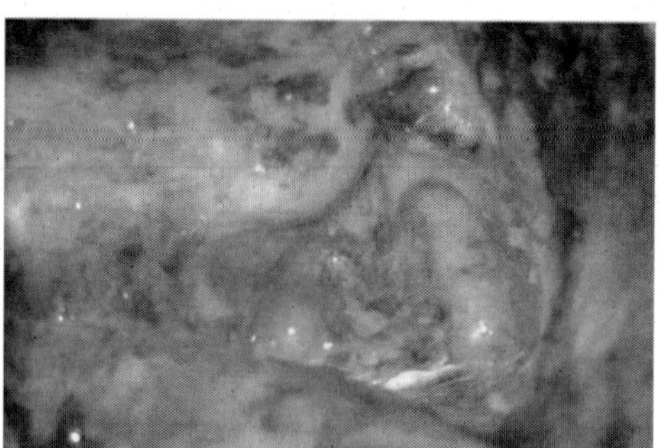

Figure 8. End of the approach: the internal auditory canal is skeletonized, and the dura exposed. The intrameatal tumor is under view, the bony canal of the superior vestibular nerve is drilled. The nerve will be further exposed and posteriorly reversed to expose the facial nerve at the fundus.

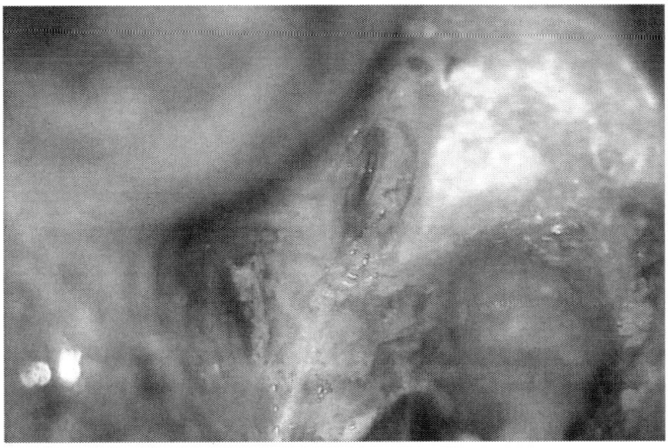

Figure 9. The positive identification of the facial nerve at the fundus is possible after reversing the superior vestibular nerve.

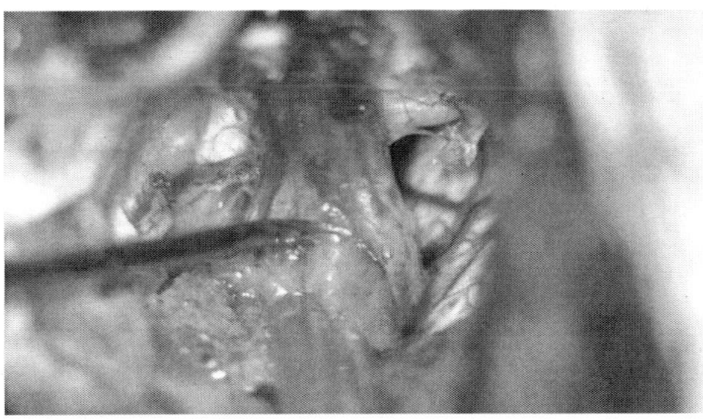

Figure 10. The dissection of the tumor begins proximally from the facial nerve at its root, then peripherically to the fundus, joining the two directions. This to minimize traction on the nerve. In the presented case, the cochlear and facial nerve are both preserved, allowing the feasibility of cochlear nerve implantation after the translabyrinthine approach.

ACKNOWLEDGMENTS

My acknowledgements are for all the oto-neurosurgical group of Padova, to the Otolaryngologist A. Martini, the Neurosurgeons D. d'Avella and L. Denaro.

REFERENCES

[1] Committee on Hearing and Equilibrium guidelines for the evaluation of hearing preservation in acoustic neuroma (vestibular schwannoma). American Academy of Otolaryngology-Head and Neck Surgery Foundation, INC. *Otolaryngol. Head Neck Surg.*, 1995; 113:179 - 80.

[2] Kanzaki, J., Tos, M., Sanna, M. et al. New and modified reporting systems from the consensus meeting on systems for reporting results in vestibular schwannoma. *Otol. Neurotol.*, 2003; 24:642,8.

[3] Stangerup, S. E., Caye-Thomasen, P. Epidemiology and natural history of vestibular schwannomas. *Otolaryngol. Clin. North Am.*, 2012 Apr.; 45(2):257 - 68.

[4] Brackmann, D. E., Cullen, R. D., Fisher, L. M. Facial nerve function after translabyrinthine vestibular schwannoma surgery. *Otolaryngol. Head Neck Surg.*, 2007; 136:773 - 7.

[5] Marchioni, D., Carner, M., Soloperto, D., Bianconi, L., Sacchetto, A., Sacchetto, L., Masotto, B., Presutti, L. Expanded transcanal transpromontorial approach: a novel surgical technique for cerebellopontine angle vestibular schwannoma removal. *Otolaryngol. Head and Neck Surg.*, 2018; 158:710 - 715.

[6] Coker, N. J., Jenkins, H. A., Fisch, U. Obliteration of the middle ear and mastoid cleft in subtotal petrosectomy: indications, technique, and results. *Ann. Otol. Rhinol. Laryngol.*, 1986; 95:5 - 11.

[7] Miller, T., Lau, T., Vasan, R. et al. Reporting success rates in the treatment of vestibular schwannomas: are we accounting for the natural history? *J. Clin. Neurosci.*, 2014; 21:914 - 8.

[8] Marston, A. P., Jacob, J. T., Carlson, M. L., Pollock, B. E., Driscoll, C. L. W., Link, M. J. Pretreatment growth rate as a predictor of tumor control following Gamma Knife radiosurgery for sporadic vestibular schwannoma. *J. Neurosurg.*, 2017; 127:380 - 387.

[9] Zanoletti, E., Cazzador, D., Faccioli, C. et al. Multi-option therapy vs observation for small acoustic neuroma: hearing-focused management. *Acta Otorhinolaryngol. Ital.*, 2018; 38(4):384 - 392.

[10] Zanoletti, E., Mazzoni, A., Martini, A. et al. Surgery of the lateral skull base: a 50-year endeavour. *Acta Otorhinolaryngol. Ital.*, 2019; 39(SUPPL.1):S1 - S146.

[11] Carlson, M. L., Vivas, E. X., McCracken, D. J. et al. Congress of Neurological Surgeons Systematic Review and Evidence-Based Guidelines on Hearing Preservation Outcomes in Patients with Sporadic Vestibular Schwannomas. *Neurosurgery,* 2018; 82.2:E35 - E39.

[12] Kirchmann, M., Karnov, K., Hansen, S. et al. Ten-year follow-up on tumor growth and hearing in patients observed with an intracanalicular vestibular schwannoma. *Neurosurgery,* 2017; 80: 49 - 56.

[13] Régis, J., Carron, R., Park, M. C., Soumare, O., Delsanti, C., Thomassin, J. M., Roche, P. H. Wait-and-see strategy compared with proactive Gamma Knife surgery in patients with intracanalicular vestibular schwannomas: clinical article. *J. Neurosurg.,* 2013; 119 Suppl.:105 - 11.

[14] Baschnagel, A. M., Chen, P. Y., Bojrab, D., Pieper, D., Kartush, J., Didyuk, O., Naumann, I. C., Maitz, A., Grills, I. S. Hearing preservation in patients with vestibular schwannoma treated with Gamma Knife surgery. *J. Neurosurg.,* 2013; 118:571 - 8.

[15] Mazzoni, A., Zanoletti, E., Denaro, L., Martini, A., Avella, D. Retrolabyrinthine Meatotomy as Part of Retrosigmoid Approach to Expose the Whole Internal Auditory Canal: Rationale, Technique, and Outcome in Hearing Preservation Surgery for Vestibular Schwannoma. *Oper. Neurosurg.,* (Hagerstown). 2018; 14:36 - 44.

[16] Zanoletti, E., Mazzoni, A., d'Avella, D. Hearing preservation in small acoustic neuroma: observation or active therapy? Literature review and institutional experience. *Acta Neurochir.,* (Wien). 2019; 161: 79 - 8.

[17] Falcioni, M., Fois, P., Taibah, A., Sanna, M. Facial nerve function after vestibular schwannoma surgery. *J. Neurosurg.,* 2011; 115: 820 - 6.

In: Vestibular Schwannoma
Editors: Francesco Dispenza et al.
ISBN: 978-1-53617-191-4

Chapter 7

THE ENLARGED TRANSLABYRINTHINE APPROACH

Maurizio Falcioni, Ilaria Iaccarino, Federica Canzano and Filippo Di Lella
ENT and Otoneurosurgical Department,
Parma University Hospital, Italy

ABSTRACT

The translabyrinthine approach (TLA) is a transpetrosal surgical approach to the cerebellopontine angle (CPA). In this approach the mastoid and posterior labyrinth are removed in order to expose the middle and posterior fossa dura and the internal auditory canal (IAC) lying immediately medial to the labyrinth itself. The idea behind the approach is to take advantage of the medial extension of the temporal bone in order to reach the CPA through the shortest route and with no or only minimal cerebellar manipulation. Theoretically the enlarged TLA allows removal of posterior fossa neoplasm of any dimensions; however, some anatomical variations of the temporal bone may require appropriate management.

Introduction and Historical Details

The translabyrinthine approach (TLA) is a transpetrosal surgical approach to the cerebellopontine angle (CPA). In this approach the mastoid and posterior labyrinth are removed in order to expose the middle and posterior fossa dura and the internal auditory canal (IAC) lying immediately medial to the labyrinth itself. Panse was credited for the first theoretical description of approaching the IAC after a labyrinthectomy in 1904; he traced his conclusions in his clinicopathologic report on temporal bone serial sections of a patient with a vestibular schwannoma. It was Quix in 1911, however, who firstly attempted tumor removal through this approach; he performed a radical mastoidectomy with facial nerve sacrifice and removed a tumor from the IAC after labyrinthectomy. Due to the fierce opposition by neurosurgeons like Cushing and Dandy, the approach was abandoned for more than half a century. It was only with William House in the 1960's that the TLA returned into surgical practice; House introduced the use of high speed drills of and binocular microscope for temporal surgery and became the first neurotologist able to deal with all the problems related with this approach (safe bone removal, facial nerve preservation) and with the CPA surgery (exposure, cerebellar retraction, hemorrhage). Since then, and with further modifications and ameliorations, the TLA became the workhorse of the neurotologist dealing with vestibular schwannoma surgery.

Surgical Concept

The idea behind the approach is to take advantage of the medial extension of the temporal bone in order to reach the CPA through the shortest route and with no or *only* minimal cerebellar manipulation (Figure 1). Following this main concept, every millimeter of bone removed slightly improves the intradural access.

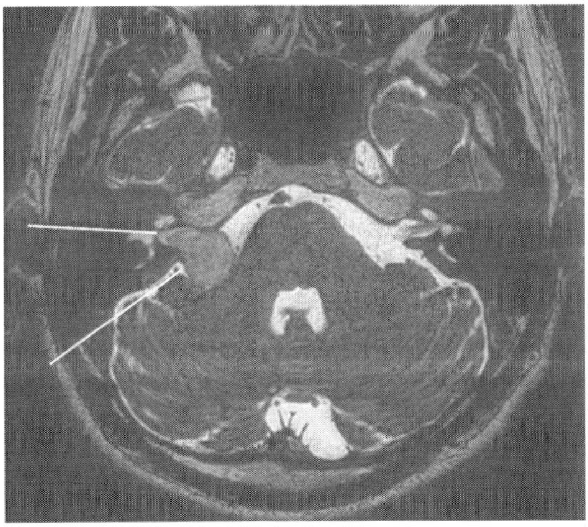

Figure 1. MRI showing the translabyrinthine route to reach the IAC/CPA.

PREOPERATIVE DETAILS

a. Magnetic resonance imaging (MRI) scans are reviewed and should be available in the operating room; the side of the surgery should always be checked together with the patient before starting preparation.
b. The hairs are shaved 7 cm posterior and 4 cm superior to the pinna with the patient awake in the anesthesia room.
c. After anesthesia induction and orotracheal intubation a nasogastric tube is placed and secured. It will help the first hours after the anesthesia, while the patient is not completely awake, to protect the airways from inhaling his/her own gastric fluids.
d. The patient is placed in the supine position with the head rotated toward the contralateral shoulder; care should be placed not to force rotation as this could compress contralateral internal jugular vein system and reduce cerebral venous blood flow. Sufficient space should be left for the surgeons' forearm to rest on the operating table both in the posterior and superior aspects of the

field. Care should be placed in securing the patient to the table as rotation of this latter is frequently required.

e. Electromyographic needles for monitoring of facial nerve muscles are positioned. Four main muscle groups are monitored, i.e., frontalis, orbicularis oculi and oris, and mentalis muscles.

f. Local anesthesia plus epinephrine is injected in the retroauricular area 10 minutes before skin incision.

g. Abdominal region is prepared and subsequently covered; the umbilical region and iliac spines should be easily identifiable as landmarks for the assistant surgeon when abdominal fat has to be harvested.

Surgical Technique

a. Soft tissues are incised in layers, to reduce risk of postoperative cerebrospinal fluid (CSF) leak. A retroauricular C-shaped skin incision is performed, starting 1 cm superior to the attachment of the pinna, running 4 cm behind the postauricular sulcus and extending just below the tip of the mastoid. An anteriorly based flap including skin and subcutaneous tissue is developed, taking care not to tear the temporalis fascial layer. Fascia will provide to the layer the strength to secure a watertight closure at the end of the procedure.

b. Myo-periosteal tissues are divided using a T shaped incision down to the underlying bone. The short arm of the T incision starts about 1 cm above the projection of the external auditory canal (EAC) and is extended posteriorly and slightly inferiorly. The long arm is located about 2 cm posterior to the EAC and extends at the level of the mastoid tip. Myo-periosteal incisions should not reach the skin, to reduce possibilities of CSF leak. The 3 flaps are carefully raised from the bone in a sub-periosteal plane with a large raspatory, with uttermost care in preserving fascial and periosteal integrity. After elevation, stay sutures (using large silk or nylon threads) are placed over the superior and posterior flaps. Elastic hooks are used for retraction of the skin, the auricle and anterior muscular flap. Stay sutures and hooks help in bleeding control and reduce the need for retractors avoiding additional unnecessary depth to the surgical field. When elevating the posterior flap bleeding from the emissary vein(s) may be controlled with bone wax or diamond burr. During elevation of the myo-periosteal layer the posterior border of the digastric groove and digastric muscle should be identified.

c. An extended mastoidectomy is performed. The middle fossa dural plate and sigmoid sinus are identified and skeletonized. The posterior fossa dural plate is identified both anterior and posterior to the sigmoid sinus.
d. The antrum is widely opened till incus visualization and the posterior wall of the EAC is thinned. The digastric ridge is identified in the posterior half of the mastoid tip and followed anteriorly.
e. The third portion of the facial nerve (FN) should now be identified. Surgical landmarks are represented by lateral semicircular canal (LSC) at the level of the second genu and the anterior extremity of the digastric ridge at the stilomastoid foramen. A cutting burr under constant irrigation is used parallel to the presumed course of the nerve. Once identified the nerve should be skeletonized with a diamond burr, but not uncovered.
f. Any mastoid emissary vein(s) should be addressed before skeletonization of dural structures. The vein(s) are uncovered distally and followed close to the sigmoid sinus using a diamond burr of appropriate size. After removal of the last shell of bone it is progressively bipolarly coagulated. In case of severe bleeding, the bony shell still present all around the sigmoid sinus allows an easy packing of the proximal vein stump.
g. Labyrinthectomy may be performed before sinus and dural uncovering or immediately after, depending on surgeon's confidence and mastoid pneumatization (in contracted mastoids it

is more comfortable to uncover the sinus and dura before labyrinthectomy). The LSC and posterior semicircular canal are blue-lined and subsequently opened, with careful identification and preservation of the medial aspects of their ampullary endings. After identification of the common crus, the superior canal is opened and its ampulla preserved as well.

h. The medial walls of the ampullary endings of the LSC and superior semicircular canal (SSC) are left in place, in order to protect the facial nerve in its labyrinthine segment. The vestibule is widely opened in its posterior aspect. Optimal exposure of the vestibule requires careful skeletonization of the medial aspect of the second genu of the FN.
i. Skeletonization and uncovering of the sigmoid sinus starts from its dome along its major axis and progressively extends anteriorly and posteriorly. The largest diamond burr is used under continuous irrigation to avoid thermal injury to the sinus; care should be taken to avoid as much as possible the use of bipolar coagulation on the vessel walls, to reduce the risk of thrombosis. It is not mandatory to fully uncover the sinus. The aim of the bone removal is to allow the surgeon to depress easily the sinus by means of the suction-irrigator, so the last tiny shell of bone may be left in place. Once the sinus has been uncovered the bone removal is extended to the retrosigmoid posterior fossa dura for 1 cm.
j. Dura of the middle fossa is then uncovered using a large diamond burr under continue irrigation and elevators. Low intensity bipolar coagulation may be used to control bleeding and to shrink the dura, providing additional extension of the approach.
k. Once the sigmoid sinus and the retrosigmoid dura have been uncovered, the presigmoid bone is addressed and skeletonized. The posterior fossa dura is detached from the bone with a large septal elevator and cottonoids. Once the cleavage plane has been established a large neurosurgical osteotome may be used to remove the bony surface already separated from the dura. In case of very thin dura this step is better achieved with the diamond burr. The

endolymphatic sac and duct are identified, with the duct running medially to the posterior semicircular canal.

l. Bone removal progresses inferiorly and the jugular bulb (JB) is identified medial to the third portion of the FN. Drilling of bone between the distal part of sigmoid sinus and the posterior aspect of the jugular bulb requires extreme care and should be performed with a diamond burr in order not to injure the vessel wall, extremely fragile at this level.
m. Dissection continues with transection of the endolymphatic duct with a micro blade after bipolar coagulation. This allows further retraction of posterior fossa dura, necessary to approach the medial part of the IAC.
n. Skeletonization of the IAC is achieved following the dura of its posterior wall, identified medial to the vestibule, the only landmark available.
o. To correctly expose the IAC, the bone inferior and superior to the canal should be removed to uncover 270° of its circumference. Superiorly there are no obstacles between middle fossa dura and the superior aspect of the canal, but care is taken to avoid injury to the FN in proximity of the fundus. Inferiorly to the IAC the cochlear aqueduct is encountered supero-medial to the jugular bulb. Opening of the cochlear aqueduct allows CSF leakage and posterior fossa decompression (in large tumors the aqueduct may be obliterated by the tumor itself). Drilling should not be extended inferior to the aqueduct to avoid injury to the glossopharyngeal nerve, lying immediately medial and anterior to it.
p. Once the IAC has been completely skeletonized the last shell of bone is removed with a micro dissector. Final drilling at the level of the fundus allows identification of the transverse crest, separating the inferior vestibular nerve inferiorly from the superior vestibular nerve superiorly (Figure 2).
q. Identification of the labyrinthine part of the FN should be now performed. With a fine diamond burr, the superior vestibular nerve is followed laterally, where it continues as the superior ampullary

nerve to the ampulla of the lateral canal. This nerve is separated from the FN at the level of the funds by a vertical bony crest, named Bill's bar after William House original description.

r. Dissection of the superior ampullary nerve from the bone with a 90 degree micro-hook is performed in a lateral to medial direction, to allow safe identification of the lateral part of the intrameatal FN. This latter lies immediately anterior to the superior ampullary nerve and in its lateral part is protected by the Bill's bar.
s. After identification of the FN and establishment of a clear cleavage plane, the inferior vestibular nerve is transected at the fundus of the IAC and reflected medially. A small piece of gelatin sponge is then placed at this level to protect the facial nerve.
t. Before posterior fossa dural opening, care is taken to close any communication between the mastoidectomy area and the middle ear, to reduce the risk of postoperative CSF leak. The incus is removed and the aditus is obliterated with periosteum. Perifacial and apical air cells are closed using bone wax.
u. After complete hemostasis is obtained, the posterior fossa dura may be opened. Bipolar coagulation is performed on the planned lines of incisions. The dura is usually opened immediately anterior to the sigmoid sinus using microsurgical scissors. After opening of the dura, a neurosurgical cottonoid is inserted and used to protect the medially lying cerebellum. An anteriorly based dural flap is progressively created, with the incisions running respectively just inferior to the superior petrosal sinus and superior to the jugular bulb.
v. Tumor removal is then performed.
w. At the end of the procedure, after completion of hemostasis, the cavity is obliterated with thin and long strips of abdominal fat, entering the CPAin layers, in order to close the dural defect in a cork-like fashion. The myo-periosteal layer is then closed using resorbable sutures, and the skin and subcutaneous tissue are closed in layers.

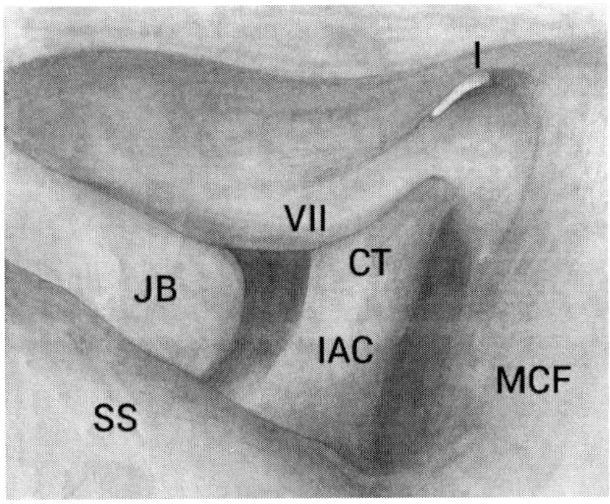

Figure 2. Schematic drawing of a standard translabyrinthine approach. I: incus; VII: facial nerve; JB: jugular bulb; SS: sigmoid sinus; MCF: middle cranial fossa; IAC: internal auditory canal; CT: cresta trasversalis.

Anatomical Variations with Surgical Implications

Theoretically the enlarged TLA allows removal of posterior fossa neoplasm of any dimensions; however, some anatomical variations of the temporal bone may require appropriate management or, in rare occasions, modification of the approach itself or combinations with other approaches. In case of significant anatomical variations, the possibility to adopt alternative approaches (as the retrosigmoid approach) should be considered and discussed with the patient.

- Anteriorly placed sigmoid sinus.
  - Sigmoid sinus position may vary in each individual depending on its development and mastoid pneumatization. An anteriorly placed sigmoid sinus is a frequent finding in temporal bone surgery, but appropriate management usually allows sufficient space to be gained in order to safely operate in the CPA. MRI

scans should always be checked to determine the size and possible dominance of the sigmoid sinus/JB complex on each side. In case of dominant sinus, maneuvers should be done with utmost and extreme care to avoid traumatic injury or thrombosis of the sinus itself. In case of an anteriorly placed sinus, the dura of the posterior fossa should be completely uncovered 2 to 3 cm posterior to the sinus. Once completely uncovered from bone, sinus and dura may be gently compressed by the instruments to approach the CPA.

- Low middle fossa dura
  - During bone removal, middle fossa dura is widely uncovered. In the rare cases of a low lying middle fossa dura, it may protrude in the surgical field and be possibly injured while drilling. Mild bipolar coagulation of the dura surface produces a shrinking of the dura itself and a consistent increase of the available surgical room.
- High riding jugular bulb

Various anomalies have been described regarding the JB; it may have an anomalous superior (high riding JB), lateral or anterior course, be partially or totally uncovered from bone into the middle ear cleft (dehiscent JB), or present a focal outpouching (JB diverticulum). These anomalies may combine each other or present as isolated findings. High riding JB is a common anomaly with a reported incidence up to 7% of cases, while JB dehiscence and JB diverticula are rarer findings. During TLA, a high riding JB, as well as JB diverticulum, may hamper surgical maneuvers around the IAC (Figure 3) and obstruct the view of the lower cranial nerve areas when working intradurally. Surgical manipulation of the JB may be performed in these cases; before attempting manipulation of the JB it is however mandatory to evaluate the MR images. A dominant sigmoid sinus/JB complex should not be posed at risk of rupture and alternative approaches should be considered (i.e., retrosigmoid or combination of TLA and retrosigmoid approaches). In fact, in the retrosigmoid approach the presencc of a high riding JB/diverticulum represents an obstacle only when treating the intracanalicular portion of the lesion.

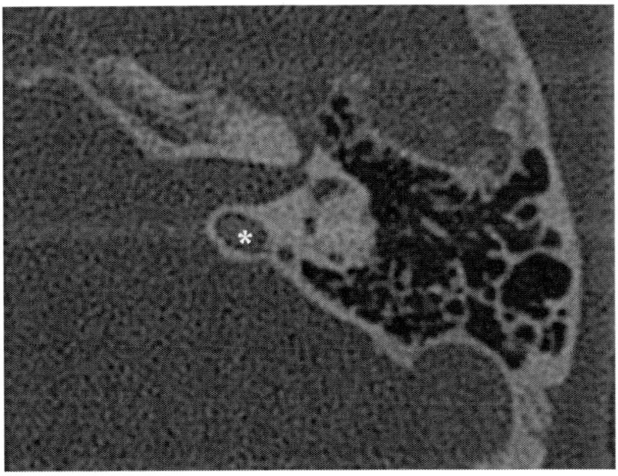

Figure 3. High jugular bulb (*) obstructing the lateral access to the IAC.

When from preoperative images it is deemed safe to manipulate the JB, it can be skeletonized using an adequate diameter diamond burr. JB treatment should be performed before dural opening, in order not to risk any bleeding entering the CPA. After skeletonization, the dome is uncovered from the bone and it is progressively dissected from its wall using an elevator. Surgicel is then used to downward compress the bulb; Surgicel is then kept in place with bone wax. Care should be taken to avoid tearing of the bulb wall as well as excessive compression of the bulb itself, because it may lead to postoperative thrombosis. After sufficient space is obtained, drill work around the IAC may be continued as usual.

Modifications of the standard technique:

a. Transapical extension.

Transapical Extension is an antero-medial extension of the enlarged TLA in which the IAC is drilled for 320° or 360° of its circumference. Usual dissection of the IAC requires exposure of more than half its circumference to safely manage the FN in its meatal portion. If control of the intradural area above and below the IAC is required (i.e., in large tumors extending to the trigeminal or lower cranial nerve area) the IAC may be dissected for around 320 degrees of its diameter (transapical extension type I). When anterior extension of the tumor is present, with need to control the prepontine cistern a complete dissection of the IAC may be performed (transapical extension type II), that allows mobilization of its contents using the suction irrigator. However, to completely achieve this target a favorable anatomy (high pneumatized temporal bone) is necessary.

b. Combination with subtotal petrosectomy.

Combination of the subtotal petrosectomy with the TLA may be indicated in different situations. In these cases, the EAC is closed in a blind sac fashion. The medial EAC skin is detached from the bone and removed in one piece together with the tympanic membrane and the malleus, after incus removal and section of the tensor tympani tendon. Care should be taken not to leave skin remnants in the area of the EAC or the annulus to avoid postoperative iatrogenic cholesteatoma. After tympanic membrane removal the posterior wall of the EAC is drilled and lowered to the level of the mastoid segment of the FN. The hypotimpanic and zygomatic root cells are removed and the mucosa of the middle ear cavity is bipolarly coagulated at low intensity. The Eustachian tube is then closed using cartilage fragments, periosteum and fibrin glue. The procedure may then be continued as usual.

In presence of extremely pneumatized temporal bone combination of subtotal petrosectomy with TLA allows reduction of the risk of CSF leak. In these cases, CSF may communicate with the tympanic cavity through the periantral, perifacial and hypotimpanic air cells. Occlusion of the Eustachian tube orifice offers an additional barrier against CSF rhinorrea.

In contracted mastoids, on the contrary, combination with subtotal petrosectomy enhances the available working room, the working angle and the light into the surgical field (Figure 4).

Finally, in presence of lesions extending posteriorly into the CPA, the subtotal petrosectomy improves the antero-posterior angle of approach eliminating the obstacle represented by the EAC.

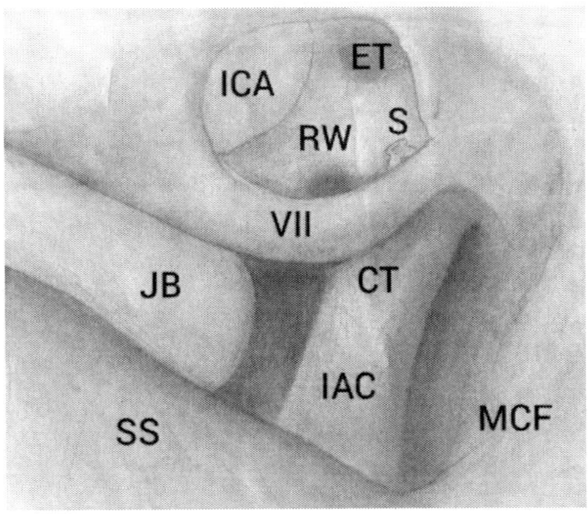

Figure 4. Schematic drawing of a standard translabyrinthine approach combined with a subtotal petrosectomy. VII: facial nerve; JB: jugular bulb; SS: sigmoid sinus; MCF: middle cranial fossa; S: stapes; RW: round window; ET: Eustachian tube; ICA: internal carotid artery.

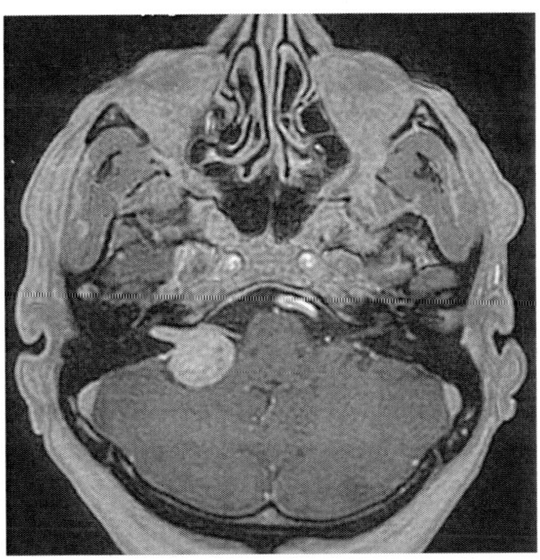

Figure 5. MRI showing a medium size vestibular schwannoma.

The disadvantages of combining the subtotal petrosectomy with TLA are represented by a longer working time (30-40 minutes), and the impossibility to achieve a watertight suture of the myo-periosteal layer at the end of the surgery, due to the missing tissue in the area previously occupied by the EAC. This can imply a higher risk of subcutaneous accumulation of CSF (usually requiring simple aspiration and compressive bandage) or cutaneous CSF leakage (sometime requiring a revision surgery).

INDICATIONS

Taking into account the complete loss of the hearing induced by the TLA and in agreement with the surgeon philosophy, presently indications for the approach may be the following:

- Acoustic neurinoma with poor preoperative hearing;
- Acoustic neurinoma larger than 1-1,5 cm in the CPA (Figure 5), where the possibilities of hearing preservation are extremely few;
- Other CPA tumors with poor chances of hearing preservation;
- temporal bone lesions with invasion of the posterior labyrinth/IAC, often in combination with other approaches (petrous bone cholesteatoma, paragangliomas, endolymphatic sac tumors, etc.).

ADVANTAGES

The following are the main advantages of TLA, when compared to the retrosigmoid approach:

- Complete control of the fundus of the IAC and with proximal identification of the FN in the lateralmost portion of its intrameatal segment;

- Shorter distance from surgeon to tumor;
- Direct access to the lateral cistern for CSF evacuation and reduction of intracranial pressure;
- Easy and fast decompression of the posterior fossa in case of postoperative intradural bleeding, by means of sutures removal and fat extraction;
- No/minimal cerebellar manipulation due to the approach;
- Direct access to large tumors for initial debulking without cerebellar manipulation, especially in presence of preoperative intracranial hypertension.

Disadvantages

The following are the main disadvantages of TLA, when compared to the retrosigmoid approach:

- Complete hearing loss;
- Technically more difficult and time demanding approach;
- Narrower approach, especially if not performed correctly;
- The available surgical room, even if the approach is correctly performed, heavely depends on individuals' anatomy.

References

Aslan, A., Falcioni, M. et al. The cochlear acqueduct: an important landmark in lateral skull base surgery. *Otolaryngol. Head Neck Surgery*, 118:532-6; 1998.

Friedman, R. A., Brackmann, D. E., van Loveren, H. R., & Hitselberger, W. E. Management of the Contracted Mastoid in the Translabyrinthine Removal of Acoustic Neuroma. *Archives of Otolaryngology - Head and Neck Surgery*, 123(3), 342-344; 1997.

Gerlings, P. G. *Atlas of the Histopathology of Ear Tumors*. Utrecht, The Netherlands: Bunge Scientific Publishers, 117-8; 1979.

Glasscock, M. E., Hays, J. W. The translabyrinthine removal of acoustic and other cerebellopontine angle tumors. *Ann. Otol. Rhinol. Laryngol.*, 82: 415-27, 1973.

House, W. F. Transtemporal bone microsurgical removal of acoustic neuromas: report of cases. *Arch. Otolaryngol.*, 80: 617-67; 1964.

Nguyen-Huynh, A. T., Jackler, R. K. et al. The aborted early history oh the translabyrinthine approach: a victim of suppression or technical pramaturity? *Otol. Neurotol.* 28: 269-279, 2007.

Naguib, M., Saleh, E. et al. The enlarged translabyrinthine approach for removal of large vestibular shwannomas. *J. Laryngol. Otol.* 108:545-50, 1994.

Panse, R. Ein Gliom des Acusticus [A glioma of the acoustic]. *Arch. Ohrenheilkd*, 61:251-5; 1904.

Roche, P. H., Moriyama, T. et al. High jugular bulb in the translabyrinthine approach to the cerebellopontine angle: anatomical considerations and surgical management. *Acta Neurochir.* (Wien). 148(4): 415-20, 2006.

Saleh, E. A., Aristegui, M. et al. Management of the high jugular bulb in the translabyrinthine approach. *Otolaryngol. Head Neck Surg*. 110(4): 397-9,1994.

Sanna, M., Saleh, E. et al. Atlas of microsurgery of the lateral skull base. *Thieme*, 2nd edition; 2007.

Sanna, M., Jain, Y. et al. Facial nerve grafting in the cerebello-pontineangle. *Laryngoscope*. 114:782-5, 2004.

Sanna, M., Russo, A. et al. Enlarged translabyrinthine approach for the management of large and giant acoustic neuromas: a report of 175 consecutives cases. *Ann. Otol. Rhinol. Laryngol*. 113:319-28, 2004.

Sanna, M., Saleh, E. et al. Identification of facial nerve in the translabyrinthine approach: an alternative technique. *Otolaryngol. Head Neck Surgery.* 124:105-6, 2001.

Sanna, M., Taibah, A. et al. Perioperative complication of acoustic neuroma (vestibular shwannoma) surgery. *Otol. Neurotol*. 25:379-86, 2004.

In: Vestibular Schwannoma
Editors: Francesco Dispenza et al.
ISBN: 978-1-53617-191-4

Chapter 8

THE RETROSIGMOID APPROACH: FROM THE MICROSURGICAL ANATOMY TO THE SURGERY

Francesca Graziano*, *Enrico Lo Bue*, *Lara Brunasso*, *Alessia Lombardo*, *Rosario Maugeri* and *Domenico G. Iacopino
Neurosurgical Clinic, AOUP "Paolo Giaccone",
Post Graduate Residency Program in Neurosurgery,
Department of Biomedicine Neurosciences
and Advanced Diagnostic (BiND),
School of Medicine, University of Palermo, 90127 Palermo, Italy

ABSTRACT

The retrosigmoid approach has been widely described and utilized for access to various pathologies of the posterior fossa and the cerebellopontine angle. This approach gives a better view of the CPA and allows early identification of various neurovascular structures, more complete removal of lesions, less morbidity, and better functional results in terms of cochlear and facial nerve preservation. Many authors advocate it as the procedure of choice during vestibular nerve section, microvascular decompression, surgery for vestibular schwannomas, non-acoustic tumors, or insertion of auditory brain stem implants.

1. Microsurgical Anatomy of the Cerebellopontine Angle

In skull base neurosurgery, the retrosigmoid approach has been widely described and utilized for access to various pathologies of the posterior fossa and the cerebellopontine angle [1]; thus, it was defined by Mostafa B E et al. as the keyhole to the Cerebello-Pontine Angle (CPA) [2]. The cerebellopontine angle is located between the superior and inferior limbs of the cerebellopontine fissure formed by the petrosal cerebellar surface folding around the pons and middle cerebellar peduncle [3]. This approach gives a better view of the CPA and allows early identification of various neurovascular structures, more complete removal of lesions, less morbidity, and better functional results in terms of cochlear and facial nerve preservation [2]. Surgery of the posterior fossa has evolved over the years with a shift toward a more minimally invasive approach [4]. Many variations of the technique have been described to tailor the procedure in relation to patient's pathology [5. 6]. Many authors advocate it as the procedure of choice during vestibular nerve section, microvascular decompression, surgery for vestibular schwannomas, non-acoustic tumors, or insertion of auditory brain stem implants [5. 6].

1.1. Osseus and Muscolar Relationships

When dealing with cerebellopontine angle approaches, surgeons initially confront the occipital and temporal bones and their related structures. Careful exposure, in particularly of bony sutures and others osseous prominences and depression, enables these sites to be used as important landmarks for surgical orientation and for restricted and appropriate CPA approaches (Figure 1) [7]. The occipital bone, situated at the back and lower part of the cranium, surrounds a large oval aperture, the foramen magnum, through which the cranial cavity communicates with the vertebral canal. The convex external surface of occipital bone has several prominences and lines on which the muscles of neck attack. The largest prominence, the external occipital protuberance or inion, is situated at the central portion of the external surface. A vertical ridge, the external occipital crest, descends from the inion to the midpoint of the posterior margin of the foramen magnum, with the nuchal ligament attached. Along the superior nuchal lines, which extend laterally and horizontally from the external occipital protuberance, the trapezius muscle inserts medially and the sternocleidomastoid muscle inserts laterally. The splenius capitis muscle, partially covered by the trapezius and sternocleidomastoid muscles, inserts on the lateral third of the superior nuchal line. The inferior nuchal lines run laterally from the midpoint of the crest. Below each inferior nuchal line, the rectus capitis posterior minor and major muscles are inserted, respectively, medially and laterally. The semispinalis capitis muscle inserts in the area between the superior and inferior nuchal lines and is situated, with the longissimus capitis muscle, deep to the splenius capitis and sternocleidomastoid muscle. Therefore, there are 4 muscular planes, which are from surface to depth: sternocleidomastoid and trapezius muscles; splenius capitis muscle; semispinalis capitis and longissimus capitis muscles; rectus capitis posterior minor, rectus capitis posterior major, inferior oblique and superior oblique muscles. The suboccipital triangle (SOT) is formed by 3 of the 4 muscles of the deepest plane: medially by the rectus capitis posterior major, laterally by the superior oblique muscle, and inferiorly by the inferior oblique muscle (Figure 2) [8]. The internal concave surface of occipital bone, in particularly of the squamous part, is deeply concave and has a prominence, the internal occipital protuberance, near its center. The cruciform eminence divides the endocranial surface of the occipital squama into four fossae. The internal occipital protuberance lies at the center of the cruciform eminence. The internal occipital crest is the inferior arm of the cruciform eminence. Transverse sulci form the transverse arms of the cruciform eminence. The occipital bone articulates with six bones: the two parietals, the two temporals, the sphenoid, and the atlas. The lambdoid, occipitomastoid, and parietomastoid sutures are united at the asterion and separate the occipital, parietal, and temporal bones (Figure 1) [7]. The asterion has been widely used as a landmark for all posterolateral approaches to the cranial base. Classically, the asterion has been cited as an external landmark for the transverse sigmoid junction (TSSJ). The relationship between the cranial sutures and venous sinuses can be used in surgical planning [7]. Posterior fossa craniotomies can constitute a risk of injury to the sinus complex due its location [9]. Localization of the venous sinuses, TSSJ and emissary vein is of utmost importance in the retrosigmoid approach to avoid damage to the venous structures of the region [10].

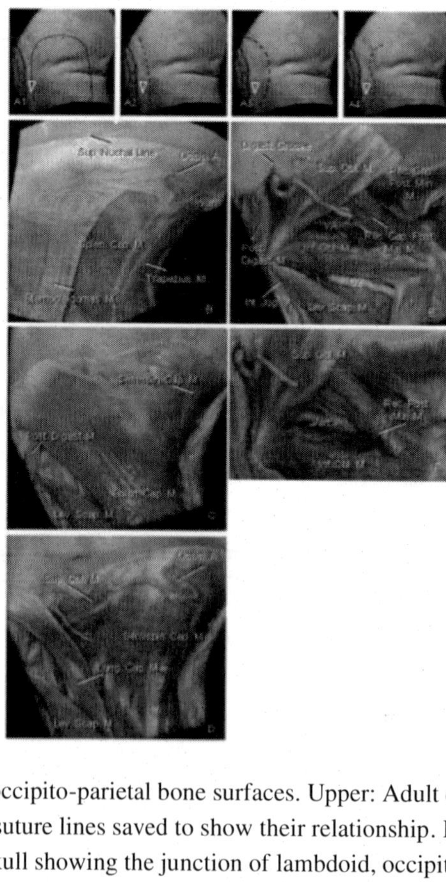

Figure 1. Temporal occipito-parietal bone surfaces. Upper: Adult cadaveric embolmed head with brain and suture lines saved to show their relationship. Lower: Lateral surface of an adult skull showing the junction of lambdoid, occipitomastoid, and parietomastoid sutures to form the asterion.

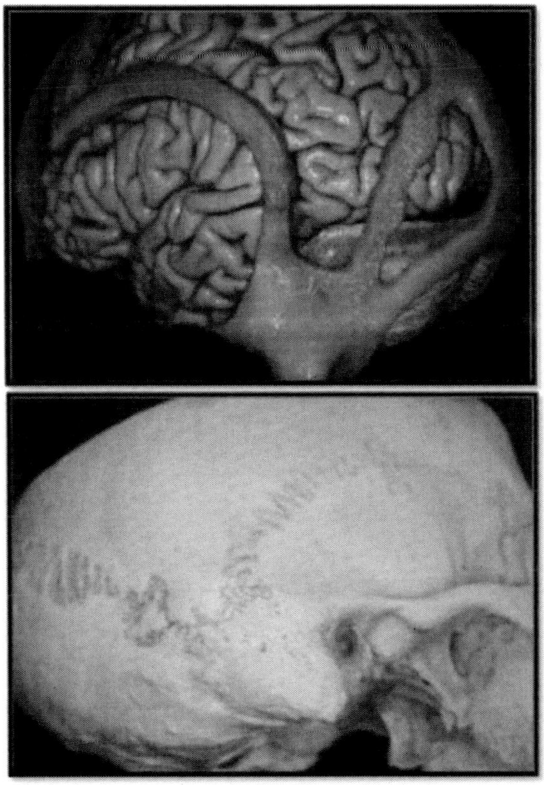

Abbreviations: sup. Superior, occip. occipital, a. artery, spleen. splenium, cap. sapitis, m. muscle, digast. digastric, obl. Oblique, rec. rectus, post. Posterior, min. minor, VA. Vertebral artery, inf. Inferior, maj. Major, int. internal, jug. Jugular, v. vein, lev. Levatoris, scap. Scapula, semispin. Semispinalis, long. Longus

Figure 2. Muscolar relationship on posterior fossa and skin incision. Adult cadaveric embolmed head. A1, A2, A3, A4: type of skin incision, reversed hockey stich, linear, C shaped, and lazy S respectively. The reversed yellow triangle indicates the mastoid tip. B, C, D, E, F: muscular planes showed in a stepwise fashion.

1.2. CPA and Its Compartments

1.2.1. CPA Upper Neurovascolar Complex

In the CPA, identification of the cranial nerves that arise from the brainstem and of their vascular relationships within the upper, middle and lower aspects of CPA cisternal space is mandatory [7]. The CPA neurovascular complex includes the pons, trigeminal nerve, supracerebellar artery (SCA) and superior petrosal veins. The most common operation directed to the upper neurovascular complex is exsposure and decompression of the posterior root of the trigeminal nerve. The posterior trigeminal root joins the brainstem about halfway between the lower and upper borders of the pons [7]. Today, it is generally agreed that the most common cause of classical trigeminal nevralgia TN is compression of the trigeminal nerve by a blood vessel, usually an artery, in the cerebellopontine cistern. This phenomenon is commonly referred to as neurovascolar conflict. A neurovascular conflict should be considered a normal neuroanatomic variant in patients with facial pain not fulfilling the TN diagnostic criteria [11]. More than one artery can compress the nerve. In a few cases the SCA will compress the rostral surface of the nerve and the anterior inferior cerebellar artery (AICA) will compress the caudal surface [7]. The SCA arises in front of the midbrain, usually from the basilar artery near the apex. It passes below the oculomotor and trochlear nerves and above the trigeminal nerve to reach the cerebellomesencephalic fissure [3].

The transverse pontine veins are the most frequent veins to compress the trigeminal nerve. The transverse veins are tributaries of the superior petrosal veins, the largest and most frequently encountered veins in the posterior fossa.

1.2.2. CPA Middle Neurovascolar Complex

The middle complex includes the AICA, pons, middle cerebellar peduncle, cerebellopontine fissure, petrosalsurface of the cerebellum and the abducens, facial and vestibulocochlear nerves. The AICA originated from the Basilar artery (98.1%) or from the vertebral artery (1.9%) as a single (92.3% of CPAs) or duplicate (7.7%) artery [12]. It courses together with the abducens, facial and vestibulocochlear nerves to reach the surface of the middle cerebellar peduncle, where it courses along the cerebellopontine fissure and terminates by supplying the petrosal surface of the cerebellum.

In most cases, the AICA passes below the facial and vestibulocochlear nerves as it encircles the brainstem. However, it may also in other cases pass above or between these nerves in its course around the brainstem. The veins on the side of the brainstem that have a predictable relationship to the facial and vestibulocochlear nerves are the veins of the pontomedullary sulcus, the veins of the cerebellomedullary fissure, middle cerebellar peduncle and cerebellopontine fissure.

Operations directed to the middle complex are for the removal of acoustic neuromas and other tumors and for the relief of hemifacial spasm. The facial and adjacent cranial nerves are the neural structures at greatest risk during acoustic neuroma removal. The facial nerve is stretched around the anterior half of the tumor capsule. The nerve infrequently is found on the posterior surface of the tumor [3].

1.2.3. CPA Lower Neurovascular Complex

The lower complex includes the posterior inferior cerebellar artery (PICA), the medulla, inferior cerebellar peduncle, cerebellomedullary fissure, suboccipital surface of the cerebellum, and the glossopharyngeal, vagus, spinal accessory and hypoglossal nerves.

The PICA arises at the medullary level from the vertebral artery, encircles the medulla, passing together with to the glossopharyngeal, vagus, spinal accessory and hypoglossal nerves to reach the surface of the inferior cerebellar peduncle. The glossopharyngeal, vagus, spinal accessory, and hypoglossal nerves arise from the medulla along the margin of the inferior olive. The PICA has a complex relationship to these nerves. The proximal part of the PICA passes around or between and often stretches or distorts the rootlets of the nerves in the lower complex. At the anterolateral medulla, the PICA passes around or between the rootlets of the hypoglossal nerve. At the posterolateral margin of the medulla, it passes between the fila of the glossopharyngeal, vagus and spinal accessory nerves. The vertebral artery courses anterior to the nerves in the lower neurovascular complex. The hypoglossal rootlets usually pass behind the vertebral artery. However, some hypoglossal rootlets infrequently pass anterior to the artery. If the vertebral artery is elongated or tortuous and courses laterally to the olive, it will stretch the hypoglossal rootless over its posterior surface. The close relationships of the PICA and vertebral artery to the glossopharyngeal and vagus nerves makes it logical to explore these relationships in glossopharyngeal neuralgia. The glossophayngeal nerve arises as one rootlet from the upper medulla, just caudal to the origin of the facial nerve. In a few cases, however, it originates as two rootlets, which can remain separated through their course to the dura. The vagus nerve arises below the glossopharyngeal nerve and is composed of multiple combinations of large and small rootlets [13]. It may be difficult to distinguish the lower vagal fibers from the upper accessory rootlets because the vagal and cranial accessory fibers usually enter the vagal meatus as a single bundle. The rootlets forming the hypoglossal nerve arise in a nucleus whose rostral portion sits deep to the hypoglossal triangle in the floor of the fourth ventricle.

2. The Retrosigmoid Approach: A Step by Step Description

2.1. Patient Positioning

The patient is placed supine or in the park-bench or sitting position [7]. Most patients are placed in a supine-oblique position, where the patient lies supine with the shoulder that is ipsilateral to the tumor elevated enough to allow the head to be turned parallel to the floor with no excessive tension on the neck [14]. A sand bag or a foam roll can be placed under the ipsilateral shoulder to minimize rotation of the neck [7]. The patient's head is rotated toward the contralateral side and is supported on a Mayfield three-point fixation device to obtain simultaneous flexion and rotation [7]. If the patient's body habitus (e.g., significant limitation of neck motion) precludes this positioning, the modified park-bench position can be considered, where the patient is placed in a lateral position with the head supported outside the surgical table by the Mayfield head holder. The dependent arm is then supported on a swing attached to the Mayfield and an axillary roll under it prevents brachial plexopathies. The ipsilateral shoulder can be taped to minimize its profile [7]. The use of sitting position has almost been abandoned because it is associated with a significant risk of air embolism, even if it offers a clean surgical field because blood and CSF drain away from it. Here, the head is slightly fixed and rotated toward the ipsilateral side [7]. The sitting position can be uncomfortable for the surgeon, leading to early interruption of the procedure. Instead, in the supine position or the modified park-bench position the operating table is turned so that the surgeon can sit behind the patient's head with his or her feet under the table. An armrest for the surgeon is also placed for the arm nearest the vertex [7].

2.2. Skin Incision

The skin incision consists of a 4–5 cm curvilinear skin incision made at the retroauricular region, and it was made to cross over the asterion at the upper third point of incision, being 1–2cm lateral to the greater occipital nerve and just medial to the lesser occipital nerves [15]. The inferior limb of the skin incision was directed laterally to avoid direct or indirect injury to the lesser occipital nerves [15]. The operative field became deeper with a linear skin incision because of the thickness of the subcutaneous tissue when retracted. Accordingly, the curvilinear incision was preferable for closing up the operative field after retracting the skin flap [15]. As the operative results have improved remarkably, the patients have begun to focus on the postoperative discomfort around the craniectomy site. One major drawback of the conventional retrosigmoid craniectomy is a possible (7–50%) postoperative headache due to the long skin incision and the large craniectomy [15, 16, 17, 18, 19, 20, 21]. Such postoperative headache may occur by adhesion of cervical musculature to dura mater with the resultant traction during neck motion, injuries to greater and/or lesser occipital nerves, or chemical meningitis by bone chips during drilling [21]. To reduce the rate of such complications and thereby improve surgical outcomes, various skin incisions and scalp flaps have been proposed as possible alternatives to the standard straight or S-shaped approach (Figure 1) [22].

To reduce postoperative headache and scalp and neck discomfort from injury to these nerves, a modified technique for a 4-cm C-shaped skin incision was developed and initially tested by Salvatore Chibbaro [23]. This modified skin incision has a medial convexity and is usually placed 8 cm laterally to the external occipital protuberance (EOP) and medially to the mastoid groove and the pinna, with the lower edge terminating 1.5-2 cm above the mastoid tip [23]. The main neural structures at risk when performing the skin incision for a minicraniotomy via retrosigmoid approach (mCRSA) are the lesser occipital nerve (LON) and the greater auricular nerve (GAN) [24, 25]: the LON runs approximately 7 cm lateral to the EOP and 3 cm medial to the mastoid process tip and provides sensorial innervation of the occipital, mastoid, and temporal regions; the GAN may have a mastoid branch running approximately 9 cm lateral to the EOP, whereas the principal trunk may be located 1cm above to the mastoid tip [24, 25]. Following a careful subperiosteal dissection, the muscle flaps are then reflected superiorly and inferiorly and retracted with stitches. After creation of a burr hole at the transverse- sigmoid sinus junction [23], a circular craniotomy approximately 2.5 cm in diameter is done, exposing the underlying dura mater, which is opened in a C-shaped fashion with the base protecting the sinus junction [23].

Asterion is a precise landmark for determining the skin incision and localizing the apex of the triangular craniectomy. It has been defined as the junction of the lambdoid, parietomastoid, and occipitomastoid sutures [27, 28], and it is easily identified as the site of slight digital depression which could be palpated through the skin behind the mastoid process at the level of zygomatic root (on the extending line from the zygomatic root to the superior nuchal line).

2.3. Bone Drilling

A retrosigmoid craniectomy usually extends from the lower margin of the transverse sinus down to the foramen magnum, behind the sigmoid sinus. In the past, the main concern during the retrosigmoid approach for CPA lesions was focused on the preservation of VIIth and VIIIth cranial nerves [15, 16, 20]. A circular craniectomy is made below asterion, overlapping the back portion of mastoid process, using a 6 mm-steel burr and a 4 mm Kerrison rongeur. The craniectomy 2 cm in width is enough to explore around V nerve or VII–VIII nerve complex and to achieve a total removal for the CPA tumors (such as vestibular schwannomas, meningiomas or cholesteatomas), while the craniectomy is a little bit enlarged downward to explore the lower CPA. A steel burr is mainly used until exposure of dura mater, while a diamond burr and Kerrison rongeurs are used for resecting the marginal inner table of the skull. The lateral border of the triangular craniectomy is approximately at the posterior margin of the sigmoid sinus, while the upper border is approximately at the inferior margin of the transverse sinus. Usually, bony removal over asterion proceeded to delineate the transverse-sigmoid junction and it is completed when the margin of the sigmoid sinus is exposed. Therefore, the final landmark of craniectomy of the subasterional approach is not exactly the asterion, but the margin of the transverse-sigmoid junction. Venous bleeding from the diploic vein, the epidural space and/or the mastoid emissary vein occurred consistently during high-speed drilling but is controlled easily using bone wax. Such hemostasis technique is indispensable for this approach (Figure 2) [15].

2.4. Dura Opening and Intradural Exposure

After the craniectomy, the dura is exposed and opened under the microscope in two possible ways. Or the dura is cut as an anteriorly based semicircular U-shaped flap, with a wide base toward the sigmoid sinus [7, 2]; this semilunar incision starts from the level of the jugular bulb and ends at the level of transverse sinus; it must be parallel and almost 1 mm posterior to the sinuses [29]. Or the dura could be also opened in a cruciate fashion and the flaps held aside with suture [30]. At the end of incisions, dura mater could be hanged anteriorly to the skin flap with sutures and stay sutures are placed on the dural edge to enhance exposure [1, 29]. The idea of making additional cuttings appears to be not necessary; furthermore, this will facilitate dura closure afterwards, at the end of surgical approach (Figure 3) [31]. When the dura cut is done, the posterior fossa dura maintains its position on the moist surface of the cerebellum, and a wet cottonoid is placed on the top of the dura to prevent drying. After its placement, it's necessary to perform intermittent irrigation of the cottonoid and the dura; this procedure ensures to avoid the desiccation of tissues [1].

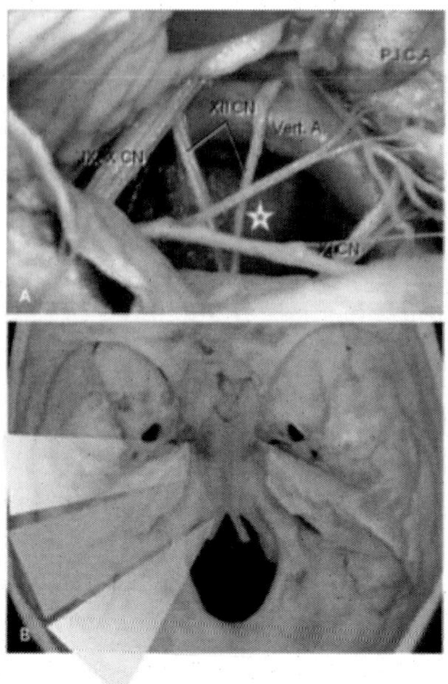

Figure 3. Intradural view and surgical approaches to posterior fossa. A. Lower exposure during retrosigmoid approach: intradural microsurgical view of the lower neurovascular complex. B. Upper view of an adult cranial fossa. The different surgical routes to the posterior fossa are showed. Yellow rectangle: Supratemporal approach-upper neurovascular complex; Green rectangle: Retrosigmoid approach- middle neurovascular complex; Light blue triangle: Lower retrosigmoid or Far lateral approach-lower neurovascular complex.

CSF Drainage Maneuvers

Neurosurgery experience showed that an important maneuver in retrosigmoid approached surgery is a sufficient drainage of CSF. After anesthesia is induced, it is appropriate to perform a CSF drain because this procedure helps minimize the retraction on the cerebellum, averts a postoperative CSF leak, decreases the pressure of the posterior fossa and facilitates the access to the lesion [7, 32]. However, in some patients, it appears to be difficult to drain the CSF because of the possibility that a fulminant cerebellar swelling may to occur after the dura mater incision; in addition, when an excessive cerebellar retraction for drainage of CSF is attempted, an unexpected cerebellar injury could be induced. Method usually used to obtain an operative corridor into the posterior fossa consists in opening the lateral cerebellomedullary cistern or the lateral cerebellopontine cistern, or cistern magna (that now results obsolete) [32]. Anyway, in alternative the placement of a lumbar drain could be a valid tool, indeed, before opening the dura mater, the lumbar drainage is opened to drain 20 to 30 cc of CSF, that is sufficient for cerebellum relaxation, than it could closed and againg opened as the surgery may require [7].

Cerebellar Retractors Placement

Retractors allow neurosurgeons to work within confined spaces, unhindered by an assistant's hand, by applying a constant force to reposition structures that would otherwise impinge on the operative line of sight [33]. However, because retractor-induced tissue edema and injury remain sources of neurosurgical morbidity, the utility of fixed retraction comes at a price; furthermore, fixed retractors require time to adjust and readjust repeatedly as the exposure demands [29].

In retrosigmoid approach, retraction of the cerebellum through retractors is seldom necessary.

The benefit of its usage is in order to obtain an adequate surgical exposure that allows the surgeon to visualize the extremely important structures in the CP angle. In particular, the direction of the application of brain spatulas for surgery admit to see different parts in the various compartments of the CP angle. Positioning retractors laterally permits to have an exposure of the middle neurovascular complex; it could be used for a lesion in the midportion of the CP angle, such as a vestibular schwannoma. Positioning retractors from top-down permits to have an exposure of the upper neurovascular complex, parallel to the superior petrosal sinus; it could be used for a microvascular decompression operation for trigeminal neuralgia. Positioning retractors from bottom-up permits to have an exposure of the lower neurovascular complex; it could be used in hemifacial spasm, because the facial nerve root exit zone is located only a few millimeters above the glossopharyngeal nerve and the PICA is commonly a compressing vessel [3]. However, in the vestibular schwannoma surgery through posterior fossa, cerebellar retraction is usually maintained for several hours, and this could provoke a cerebellar injury [29].

Because of the need to find a safe and effective solution to avoid the possibility of injury due to its utilization, now cerebellar retractors are not required in posterior fossa approaches because of refinements of the surgical and neuroanesthesia [29]. Indeed, when adequate conditions such as patient positioning, adequate anesthesia techniques, and surgical manipulations are applied in posterior fossa approach (except for neurovascular decompression and some of the acoustic neuroma surgeries), cerebellar retractors are not needed [29]. For example, a surgical manipulation, in which their usage is not required, consists in suturing the dura anteriorly over the sigmoid sinus because this maneuver could allow the maximal anterior exposure [1]. Moreover, another option is to insert a spatulum fixed by a Leyla-retractor and gain insight to the CP angle to hold (not retract!) the cerebellum [31].

2.5. Tumor Exposure and Removal

In the first moments of the dissection, when it is easiest to distinguish tumor from surrounding tissues, arachnoid adhesions are released and the cerebellum and lower cranial nerves are separated from the tumor. Once the cranial nerves have been identified, the tumor is morcellized from its core through ultrasonic aspiration, which is especially helpful when resecting the core of the tumor because it allows the removal of its smaller fragments. An important procedure during tumor removal is the monitoring of the facial nerve. If there are some evidence of its irritation, the surgeon should think about changing the area of dissection; in facts, after the facial nerve identification, it is important to perform a dissection of it from the tumor with a round knife. The facial nerve is usually displaced anteriorly against the anterior rim of the internal auditory canal, and this spot is most susceptible to injury during dissection [7]. After brain tumor removal, hemostasis could be performed using hemostat such as TachoSil, a sponge with an active yellow side coated with human thrombin and human fibrinogen. Its effect can be enhanced and supported by an autologous fibrin sealant to cover the surgical bed and to achieve dural closure, repair of dural defects, and to fill "dead spaces" with the same product [34, 35]. The microscopical approach may gain some advantages from the endoscopic technique. The application of neuroendoscopy will likely reflect less-invasive alternatives of traditional skull base approaches and may enhance the surgical view along deep or tight corridors not well visualized with the binocular microscopic view [36].

2.6. Closure Techniques

Once tumor removal is complete and hemostastis is obtained, the tack-up dural sutures applied during the dural opening phase are cut and the dura could be closed with 4-0 woven nylon suture; in order to guarantee a major stability, a patch of blood-impregnated microfibrillar collagen hemostat is layered on top of the dural closure filling the craniectomy defect [7, 1]. Another way to make duroplasty is using the autologous pericranium graft, inserting it through the defect as an underlay hourglass-shaped plug. For obtaining this, the graft harvested has to be slightly larger than the dural defect, in order to have its edges under the dural plane and then it is fixed under operative microscope magnification with separated stitches (with an "inside-to-outside" direction) to the dura mater, using a 3-

0 running silk. After that, the inserted patch was augmented with one layer of absorbable hemostats, with small pieces of surgical patches and with dural sealant [34]. In consideration of the thinness and fragility of pericranium in some population, like children, it could be another option to use ligamentum nuchae as graft; it could be more robust than pericranium, but this statement needs to be considered with caution and the understanding that this may not be true for all age groups [38]. When the duroplasty is complete, the bony defect could be filled with different materials, that reduce the risk of postoperative headache, such as: acrylic muscle, fibrin glue, wax or polymethyl methacrylate (PMMA). The muscles are then closed in layers primarily using their respective fascial planes with interrupted 2-0 woven polyglactic acid suture [1]. During closure, the aponeurotic fascia that was dissected before, could be an extra layer that helps to achieve a more hermetic closure [7, 39, 40]. The deep layer of the skin is closed with inverted, interrupted sutures, in which the staples are used to approximate the skin. Antibiotic ointment is applied to the staples and a 5x 3x 7cm island-type dressing is placed over the staple line; since this is not a pressure dressing, it can be removed the day after surgery [1].

References

[1] Venable, et al. Primary Dural Closure for Retrosigmoid Approaches. *J Neurol Surg B.*, 2017.

[2] Mostafa, BE; El Sharnoubi, M; Youssef, AM. The Keyhole Retrosigmoid Approach to the Cerebello-Pontine Angle: Indications, Technical Modifications, and Results. *Skull Base*, Volume 18, Number 6, 2008.

[3] Rhoton, AL. The Cerebellopontine Angle and Posterior Fossa Cranial Nerves by the Retrosigmoid Approach. *Neurosurgery*, 2000, 47, S93–129.

[4] Wackym, PA; King, WA; Meyer, GA; Poe, DS. Endoscopy in neuro-otologic surgery. *Otolaryngol Clin North Am*, 2002, 35, 297–323.

[5] Magnan, J; Barbieri, M; Mora, R; et al. Retrosigmoid approach for small and medium-sized acoustic neuromas. *Otol Neurotol*, 2002, 23, 141–145.

[6] Miyazaki, H; Deveze, A; Magnan, J. Neuro-otologic surgery through minimally invasive retrosigmoid approach: endoscope assisted microvascular decompression, vestibular neurotomy, and tumor removal. *Laryngoscope*, 2005, 115, 1612–1617.

[7] Bambakidis, NC; Megerian, CA; Robert, F; Spetzler, F. *Surgery of the cerebellopontine Angle*.

[8] Campero, A; Villalonga, JF; Elizalde, RL; Ajler, P. The Nuchal Lines as Anatomic Landmarks to Dissect the Muscles in the Far Lateral Approach. *World Neurosurg*, 2018, 113, 188–94.

[9] Uz, A; Ugur, HC; Tekdemir, I. Is the asterion a reliable landmark for the lateral approach to posterior fossa? *J Clin Neurosci*, 2001, 8, 146–7.

[10] da Silva, EB; Leal, AG; Milano, JB; da Silva, LFM; Clemente, RS; Ramina, R. Image-guided surgical planning using anatomical landmarks in the retrosigmoid approach. *Acta Neurochir* (Wien), 2010, 152, 905–10.

[11] Di Stadio, A; Dipietro, L; Toffano, R; Burgio, F; De Lucia, A; Ippolito, V; Garofalo, S; Ricci, G; Martines, F; Trabalzini, F; Della Volpe, A. Working memory function in children with single side deafness using a bone-anchored hearing implant: A case-control study. *Audiology and Neurotology*, (2018), 23 (4), pp. 238-244.

[12] Kim, HN; Kim, YH; Kim, GR; Park, IY; Chung, IH. Variability of the Surgical Anatomy of the Neurovascular Complex of the Cerebellopontine Angle. *Ann Otol Rhinol Laryngol*, 1990, 99, 288–96.

[13] Tarlov, IM. Structure of the nerve roots: II. Differentation of sensory from motor roots; observations on identification of function in roots of mixed cranialnerves. *Arch Neurol Psychiatry*, 1937, 37, 1338.

[14] Ojemann, RG. Retrosigmoid Approach to Acoustic Neuroma (Vestibular Schwannoma). *Neurosurgery*, vol 48, No 3, March 2001.

[15] Scorpecci, A; Massoud, M; Giannantonio, S; Zangari, P; Lucidi, D; Martines, F; Foligno, S; Di Felice, G; Minozzi, A; Luciani, M; Marsella, P. Otogenic lateral sinus thrombosis in children: proposal of an experience-based treatment flowchart. *European Archives of Oto-Rhino-Laryngology*, (2018), 275 (8), pp. 1971-1977.

[16] Fukuhara, T; Silverman, DA; Hughes, GB; Kinney, SE; Newman, CW; Sandridge, SA; et al. Vestibular nerve sectioning for intractable vertigo: efficacy of simplified retrosigmoid approach. *Otol Neurotol.*, 2002, 23, 67-72.

[17] De Stefano A., Kulamarva G., Dispenza F. Malignant paroxysmal positional vertigo. *Auris Nasus Larynx.*, 2012 Aug, 39(4), 378-82. doi: 10.1016/j.anl.2011.07.008. Epub 2011 Aug 30.

[18] Dispenza, F., DE Stefano, A., Costantino, C., Rando, D., Giglione, M., Stagno, R., Bennici, E. Canal switch and re-entry phenomenon in benign paroxysmal positional vertigo: difference between immediate and delayed occurrence. *Acta Otorhinolaryngol Ital.*, 2015 Apr, 35(2), 116-20.

[19] Dispenza, F., De Stefano, A.Vertigo in childhood: a methodological approach. *Bratisl Lek Listy.*, 2012, 113(4), 256-9. Review.

[20] Silverman, DA; Hughes, GB; Kinney, SE; Lee, JH. Technical modifications of suboccipital craniectomy for prevention of postoperative headache. *Skull Base.*, 2004, 14, 77-84.

[21] Schaller, B; Baumann, A. Headache after removal of vestibular schwannoma via the retrosigmoid approach: a long-term follow-up-study. *Otolaryngol Head Neck Surg.*, 2003, 128, 387-395.

[22] Jannetta, PJ; McLaughlin, MR; Casey, KF. Technique of microvascular decompression; technical note. *Neurosurg Focus.*, 2005, 18, E5.

[23] Salvatore, Chibbaro; et al. Retrosigmoid Approach: Investigating the Role of a C-Shaped Skin Incision and Muscle Flaps in Improving Functional Outcome and Reducing Postoperative Pain. *World Neurosurg.*, (2017).

[24] Tomasello, F; Esposito, F; Abbritti, RV; Angileri, FF; Conti, A; Cardali, SM; et al. Microvascular decompression for trigeminal

neuralgia: technical refinement for complication avoidance. *World Neurosurg.*, 2016, 94, 26-31.

[25] Lee, M; Brown, M; Chepla, K; Okada, H. Gatherwright J, Totonchi A, et al. An anatomical study of the lesser occipital nerve and its potential compression points: implications for surgical treatment of migraine headaches. *Plast Reconstr Surg.*, 2013, 132, 1551-1556.

[26] Tubbs, RS; Loukas, M; Shoja, MM; Bellew, MP; Cohen-Gadol, AA. Surface landmarks for the junction between the transverse and sigmoid sinuses: application of the "strategic" burr hole for suboccipital craniotomy. *Neurosurgery.*, 2009, 65, (6 suppl), 37-41 [discussion: 41].

[27] Bannister, LH; Berry, MM; Collins, P; Dyson, M; Dussek, JE; Ferguson, MWJ. (eds) Gray's anatomy. 38th edn. *Churchill Livingstone*, New York, 1995, 561.

[28] Aysun, Uz; Hasan Caglar Ugur, I. brahim Tekdemir. Is the asterion a reliable landmark for the lateral approach to posterior fossa? *Journal of Clinical Neuroscience*, (2001), 8(2), 146–147.

[29] Nebil, Goksu; Yildirim, A. Bayazit; Ismet, Bayramoglu; Berrin, Isik; Metin, Yilmaz; Omer, Kurtipek; Kemal, Uygur. Surgical exposure in retrosigmoid approach: do we need cerebellar retractors? *Surgical neurology*, 65, (2006), 631-634.

[30] Roberto, A; Cueva, Bill Mastrodimos. *Approach design and closure techniques to minimize cerebrospinal fluid leak after cerebellopontine angle tumor surgery.*, 26, 1176-1181, 2005, Otology & Neurotology, Inc.

[31] Marcos, Tatagiba; Florian, Roser; Martin, U. Schuhuman; Florian, H. Ebner. Vestibular schwannoma surgery via the retrosigmoid transmeatal approach. *Acta Neurochir*, (2014), 156, 421-425.

[32] Chang, Kyu Park; Sung, Ho Lee; Bong, Arm Rhee; Seok, Keun Choi. Puncture of Cerebellar Horizontal Fissure for Retrosigmoid Approach: a prospective and quantitative analysis. *Operative Neurosurgery*, 0, 1-4, 2017.

[33] Robert, F. Spetzler, Nader Sanai. The quiet revolution: retractorless surgery for complex vascular and skull base lesions. *J Neurosurg*, 116, 291-300, 2012.

[34] Graziano, F; Maugeri, R; Iacopino, DG. Intraparenchymal brain hemorrhage: "birdlime" effect usefulness. *World Neurosurg.*, (2018), 120, 598.

[35] Graziano, F; Certo, F; Basile, L; Maugeri, R; Grasso, G; Meccio, F; Ganau, M; Iacopino, DG. Autologous fibrin sealant (Vivostat (®)) in the neurosurgical practice: Intracranial surgical procedure. *Surg Neurol Int.*, 2015, May 12, 6, 77.

[36] Russo, VM; Graziano, F; Quiroga, M; Russo, A; Albanese, E; Ulm, JA. Minimally invasive supracondylar transtubercular (MIST) approach to the lower clivus. *World Neurosurg.*, (2012), 77, 5/6, 704-712.

[37] Mastronardi, L; Cacciotti, G; Caputi, F; Roberto, R; Tonelli, MP; Carpineta, E; Fukushima, T. Underlay hourglass-shaped autologous pericranium duroplasty in "key-hole" retrosigmoid approach surgery: Technical report. *Surg Neurol Int.*, 2016, Mar 10, 7, 25.

[38] Cools, MJ; Quinsey, CS; Elton, SW. Ligamentum nuchae as a graft material for duroplasty in patients with Chiari malformation type I. Published online July 13, 2018; DOI: 10.3171/2018.5.PEDS18301.

[39] Dispenza, F., Mazzucco, W., Bianchini, S., Mazzola, S., Bennici, E. Management of labyrinthine fistula in chronic otitis with cholesteatoma: Case series (2015) *EuroMediterranean Biomedical Journal*, 10 (21), pp. 255-261.

[40] Dispenza F., Battaglia A. M., Salvago P., Martines F. Determinants of failure in the reconstruction of the tympanic membrane: a case-control study. *Iranian J of Otorhinolaryngol.*, 2018, 30, 341-346.

In: Vestibular Schwannoma
Editors: Francesco Dispenza et al.
ISBN: 978-1-53617-191-4

Chapter 9

MIDDLE FOSSA APPROACH FOR VESTIBULAR SHWANNOMA: AN OVERVIEW

Rosario Maugeri[1,*], MD, PhD, Giuseppe Roberto Giammalva[2], MD, Francesca Graziano[1]MD, PhD, Teresa Somma[2], MD, Carlo Gulì[1], MD, Mariangela Pino[1], MD and Domenico Gerardo Iacopino[1] MD, PhD

[1]Department of Biomedicine, Neurosciences and Advanced Diagnostics, School of Medicine, Postgraduate Residency Program in Neurological Surgery, Neurosurgical Clinic, AOUP "Paolo Giaccone," Palermo, Italy

[2]Department of Neurosciences and Reproductive and Dental Sciences, Division of Neurosurgery, University of Naples "Federico II," Naples, Italy

[*] Corresponding Author's Email: Rosario.maugeri1977@gmail.com.

ABSTRACT

The Middle Fossa Approach (MFA) is ideally used for hearing preservation in relatively young patients with small intracanalicular VS with serviceable hearing, especially when there is lateral extension of the VS into the fundus of the IAC. MFA provides a short surgical corridor to approach the tumour with minimal manipulation of the cranial nerves VII and VIII, thus reducing the odds of cranial nerves impairment. Significant tumour extension medially into the cisternal space of the cerebellopontine angle is considered a limitation to this approach.

INTRODUCTION

Vestibular schwannomas (VS) account up to approximately 8% of all intracranial tumours. VS arise from the vestibular portions of the eighth cranial nerve, which runs in conjunction with the seventh cranial nerve through the cerebellar-pontine angle (CPA) into the internal acoustic canal (IAC), through the Obersteiner-Redlich transition zone [17, 22, 33].

The incidence is estimated to be 1.9 per 100,000 per year. Patients typically present tinnitus, imbalance, dizziness and hearing loss [29].

Various theories are related to the mechanism of hearing loss: tumour-induced pressure in the IAC, vascular compromise, cochlear hair cell loss and altered composition of fluids within the inner ear.

The widespread use of magnetic resonance imaging of the brain has led to early diagnosis of VS with smaller size in patients with yet intact hearing in early stages.

Several factors contribute to the decision-making process, including hearing status, age, tumour location, and tumour size. Often the final therapeutic decision is based on patient's preference after a thorough discussion on the advantages and disadvantages of treatment options [16].

The three treatment options are envisaged for such patients: expectant observation, stereotactic radiosurgery (SRS), and microsurgery [25]. Conservative management with watchful waiting is typically reserved for small tumours in patients with minimal or no symptoms, poor overall health, or advanced age. Hearing loss in an expected outcome of conservative management over time, so most young and middle-aged patients with even minimal symptoms prefer SRS or microsurgical resection for better long-term hearing outcomes. Conventionally, SRS has been used for small tumours (<2.5 cm), tumours in older patients, and recurrent/residual VS. Initial reports suggested that SRS seems to offer better facial nerve (FN) and hearing preservation rates than corresponding microsurgical resection for such patient groups, but adequate long-term data are still missing. Microsurgery is classically reserved for symptomatic, younger patients with good overall functional performance status [25].

A multidisciplinary team approach with a neuro-otologist and a neurosurgeon is advocated in order to offer the patient the expertise of both specialties and maximizes safety and the chances for an optimal outcome. VS can typically be surgically approached by translabyrinthine, retrosigmoid, or middle fossa approach [4].

The translabyrinthine approach allows a greater exposure at the cost of hearing loss. The retrosigmoid approach is more familiar for neurosurgeons, it ensures a panoramic view of the posterior cranial fossa and it avoids the retraction of the temporal lobe; the disadvantages are limited exposure of the fundus of the IAC, late exposure of the facial nerve and a higher incidence of headaches. The retrosigmoid approach is mostly adopted when one of the goals of VS surgery is hearing preservation, which ranges from 21 to 71% through this approach [16].

The Middle Fossa Approach (MFA) is ideally used for hearing preservation in relatively young patients with small intracanalicular VS with serviceable hearing, especially when there is lateral extension of the VS into the fundus of the IAC. MFA provides a short surgical corridor to approach the tumour with minimal manipulation of the cranial nerves VII and VIII, thus reducing the odds of cranial nerves impairment. Significant tumour extension medially into the cisternal space of the cerebellopontine angle is considered a limitation to this approach [23].

MFA to the IAC and adjacent structures was developed by in 1961 in an effort to remove foci of labyrinthine otosclerosis. Although he used this approach briefly for the removal of acoustic tumours, he soon directed his efforts to the translabyrinthine approach [24].

However, further experiences demonstrated that MFA was most suitable for small tumours and that preservation of hearing and facial nerve function was possible in a significant portion of operated patients, ranging from 50% to 69% [14].

Potential prognostic indicators for hearing preservation have been widely examined. Preoperative hearing status, auditory brainstem response, tumour size and intraoperative anatomic findings have all been evaluated as potential prognostic indicators in most reports [1, 3, 15, 16].

Preservation of the FN is one of the main goals in VS surgery to prevent disfiguring and disabling facial palsy, which severely affects the quality of life of these patients [10].

Through MFA, few reliable anatomic landmarks are revealed during exposure of the IAC, and their position is difficult to be identified. Therefore, there is a possibility of nerve damaging; in particular the greater superficial petrosal nerve and the facial nerve lying between the tumour and surgeon.

In various series, good FN outcome (HB grade I/II) after MFA has been achieved in 88%-100% of patients [3, 15, 25, 26].

The availability of superior microscopes, safer highspeed drills, better haemostatic agents, autologous glues, an endoscope assisted strategy and intraoperative neuromonitoring shifted the goals of MFA in VS surgery from preserving life to preserving FN function and hearing [11, 12].

INDICATION

The primary indications for the middle fossa approach are small acoustic tumours, with less than 5 mm extension into the cerebellopontine angle, and good preoperative hearing. The MFA provides complete exposure of the contents of the IAC, thus allowing the removal of lesions which are laterally placed without the need for blind dissection [14].

As all surgical approaches for VS resection, MFA presents both advantages and disadvantages. As advantages, MFA allows the highest hearing preservation rates, it reduces the incidence of postoperative headache, it improves the exposure of the lateral IAC as compared with retrosigmoid approach, and it allows a complete bone removal prior to dural opening. As disadvantages, MFA provides a limited access to the posterior cranial fossa, its employment is influenced by tumour size and it entails a higher risk of postoperative facial nerve weakness [6].

SURGICAL ANATOMY

The surgical anatomy of the temporal bone for the middle fossa approach is complex, since landmarks are not as apparent as with other approaches through the temporal bone. In this case, laboratory dissection is useful for the surgeon to become familiar with the anatomy of the temporal bone aproached from above [14].

The floor of the middle fossa hosts several important structures. Rhoton et al. divided the floor with a vertical plane through the anterior border of the cochlea. Anteriorly, the Eustachian tube, tensor tympani, and petrous carotid artery from the lateral to medial lie parallel and deep to the greater superficial petrosal nerve (GSPN) in the space between the V3 division of the trigeminal nerve anteriorly and the cochlea posteriorly. The posterior part of the floor contains the bony labyrinth with three components: the cochlea, the vestibule, and superior semicircular canals (SSCs). This part is more vulnerable to injury during surgery because of the intimate relation with the lateral part of the IAC. The cochlea is located at the cochlear angle between the GSPN and the labyrinthine part of the facial nerve, just anterior to the lateral IAC fundus. The vestibule is a small cavity located in the posterolateral margin of the IAC fundus. The superior SSCs project toward the middle fossa floor and make a bony elevation known as the arcuate eminence (AE). The foramen spinosum is located just posterolateral to the foramen ovale, with the middle meningeal artery (MMA) passing through it. The GSPN originates from the geniculate ganglion (GG) and passes anteriorly in the sphenopetrosal groove beneath V3 toward the foramen lacerum and then joins the lesser petrosal nerve to form the vidian nerve in its canal. At its lateral extent, the IAC is divided into four quadrants. Bill's bar (vertical crest) separates the facial nerve in the superior-anterior quadrant from the superior vestibular nerve in the superior-posterior quadrant. The transverse crest, on the other hand, separates the superior vestibular nerve in the superior-posterior quadrant from the inferior vestibular nerve in the inferior-posterior quadrant [2].

As regards MFA, the House's technique provides direct vision of the IAC, allowing possible complete removal of tumours, while preserving hearing and facial nerve function. The technique proposed by House is to firstly identify the GSPN, then to expose the geniculate ganglion (GG), and the first genu of the facial nerve. At this point, the labyrinthine portion of the facial nerve is followed to the lateral end of the IAC. This method endangers the important structures which are closely related to the fundus of the IAC.

Later, Fisch described the method of locating the IAC, which lies at 60° degrees angle anterior to the superior semicircular canal (SSCC). However, the angle is inconstant. Garcia-Ibanez identified the IAC by bisecting the angle formed by the GSPN and the arcuate eminence. However, the arcuate eminence is not identified in all the cases and is not at the same axis with the SSCC in 48% of cases. Recently, Lan and Shiao described a new and simple method to safely identify the IAC without the risk of damaging the cochlea, facial nerve, and vestibule, by using the GSPN and the GG as the only two landmarks [18].

Image guided navigation through the temporal bone has been introduced as an accurate alternative method to localize the IAC without the need to expose the GG or the SSC.

Because of the wide variations in anatomy and small working space, no single technique can ensure avoidance of injury to important structures. In order to obtain a successful operative planning, careful dissection and a detailed understanding of the regional anatomy are necessary [13, 30].

SURGICAL TECHNIQUE

The procedure is performed in general anesthesia with endotracheal tube. The patient is positioned supine on the surgical table, whit the head fixed in a Mayfield clamp turned contralateral to the lesion so that the affected ear is as parallel as possible to the floor. Neuromonitoring for facial nerve, electromyography and auditory brainstem response are set up [6]. A lumbar spinal catheter for cerebrospinal fluid drainage is used to minimize the amount of temporal lobe retraction [31].

The surgeon is seated at the head of the table, and the anesthesiologist is at the foot. The skin incision is made in the pretragal area and it is extended superiorly in a gently curving fashion. An inferiorly based U-shaped flap is fashioned of the temporalis muscle and fascia. This flap is reflected inferiorly. Using a cutting bur, a craniotomy opening is made in the squamous portion of the temporal bone. Craniotomy extends approximately two thirds anterior and one third posterior to the external auditory canal and it is approximately 2.5 cm square. This bone flap is based on the root of the zygoma as close to the floor of the middle fossa as possible. During creation of this flap, care is taken to avoid laceration of the underlying dura [14]. Any lateral air cells which might be opened are covered with bone wax. Under magnification, the dura is elevated off the floor of the temporal fossa, posteriorly from the petrous ridge and anteriorly to identify the greater superficial petrosal nerve. The posterior to anterior dissection avoids the risk of dissecting below the greater superficial petrosal nerve and inadvertently avulsing it from the facial hiatus. Venous bleeding is commonly encountered in the region of the foramen spinosum. We avoid coagulation in this location to minimize the risk of both injury to the greater superficial petrosal nerve and interruption of any blood supply to the facial nerve that could arise from the region of the foramen spinosum. Generally, this bleeding is easily managed with gentle tamponading with one of a variety of haemostatic materials. Once the greater superficial petrosal nerve is identified, dural elevation continues to the true petrous ridge. A self-retaining brain retractor is used to maintain a visible plane of dissection. The superior semicircular canal is identified either by direct visualization or by blue-lining of the canal. Typically, the IAC bisects the angle between the course of the greater superficial petrosal nerve and the orientation of the superior semicircular canal. This angle tends to be approximately 60° from the course of the greater superficial petrosal nerve, but the anatomical relationship varies. Bone anterior and medial to the superior semicircular canal is removed to identify the dura around the porus acousticus. Bone removal continues laterally along the course of the IAC until Bill's bar, or separation of the facial nerve from the vestibular nerve, is exposed. The cochlea lies just anterior to the lateral IAC, and no attempt is made to expose it [6].

Subsequently, the dura mater of the IAC is opened at its posterior aspect to prevent accidental damage to the underlying facial nerve (FN), which lies on the anterosuperior aspect of the IAC. After the spillage of cerebrospinal fluid (CSF), the FN is identified by direct stimulation through electric probe, then a dissection of the plane of cleavage between the FN and the tumour interface is performed. In order obtain a careful dissection, sodium fluorescein, may play a role in enhancing the optical definition of the lesion [5, 7, 19]. After the anatomical and functional definition of the tumour, it is gradually removed using careful medial to lateral dissection together with debulking of the tumour mass (performed by micro-scissors or ultrasonic aspirator). Any dissection of tumour in the opposite direction (from lateral to medial) should be avoided to prevent avulsion of cochlear nerve fibres entering the lamina cribrosa laterally. Coagulation should be avoided to prevent heat transmission to the FN or auditory nerve; if neater dissection planes are needed, larger tumours should be dissected under constant irrigation [10]. Any exposed air cells are sealed off using bone wax, and dural defect is sealed by using an appropriately sized autologous fat graft harvested from the abdomen, which is reinforced by tissue glue [8, 9, 11, 12, 20, 21, 25].

The rest of the closure is done layer by layer, with closure of the muscle, fascia, galea, and skin [4].

COMPLICATIONS

Microsurgery for small acoustic neuromas through the MFA is an established method that is associated with a low complication rate [28].

Postoperative cerebrospinal fluid (CSF) leakage is a typical complication. The incidence varies from 4 to 19%. The extent of pneumatization of the petrous bone is a well-known predictor of CSF leakage. Another typical risk factor is the consistency of the dura, which is worse or more fragile in the elderly. This may lead to the rupture of the dura during its separation or retraction [27].

First treatments of CSF leak are conservative measures like bed rest, pressure dressings and i. v. antibiotics since this results in a high rate of spontaneous closure of the leakage. In case of failure of conservative management, a lumbar drainage may be placed. If these non-surgical procedures are not successful, surgical re-exploration is indicated.

The MFA requires *retraction of the temporal lobe*; therefore, injury can potentially occur (e.g., aphasia, hemiparesis, or seizure).

This elevation might come along with a compression of the auditory fields within the lobe. Several authors report of contralateral hearing loss after otologic and non-otologic intradural skull base surgery. Various mechanisms have been proposed including meningitis, ototoxicity, autoimmune reaction, vascular compromise, allergy, labyrinthine rupture from elevated intratympanic pressures, or acoustic trauma because of drill noise. Moreover, loss of hearing can be caused by the intraoperative reduction of CSF pressure, which leads to a low perilymphatic pressure and a compensatory elevation of endolymphatic pressure [32].

Intracranial haemorrhage occurs in 0.4%-2% of MFA procedures and it can present as sub- or epidural bleeding as well as bleeding of the cerebellum or brainstem. Despite this low incidence, intracranial bleedings are the most common cause of death after surgery. Intracranial haemorrhage can be promoted by the reduced CSF pressure. Extensive CSF spillage can stretch subdural veins until their rupture. This should be taken particularly into account for elderly patients in whom the dura is more fragile.

Postoperative meningitis can be either aseptic or bacterial. Most cases of postoperative meningitis are aseptic and caused by irritation of the meninges by blood, bone dust, or foreign materials. Bacterial meningitis can occur by ascension of germs, which can be promoted by CSF leakage [28].

Conclusion

The middle fossa approach is best suited for lesions situated lateral within the internal auditory canal that have limited extension into the CPA (less than 1 cm) and where hearing preservation is the goal. This approach requires a detailed understanding of the complex temporal bone anatomy with its landmarks.

Careful dissection and a detailed understanding of the regional anatomy are key elements for success.

References

[1] Aihara N, Murakami S: Enlargement of the Internal Auditory Canal and Hearing Preservation in the Middle Fossa Approach for Intracanalicular Vestibular Schwannomas. *World Neurosurg*. 84: 1950-1955, 2015 Available: http://www.ncbi.nlm.nih.gov/pubmed/26341444. Accessed 14 February 2019.

[2] Alzhrani G, Shelton C, Couldwell WT: Middle fossa approach for resection of vestibular schwannoma. *Acta Neurochir*. (Wien) 159:1023-1026, 2017 Available: http://www.ncbi.nlm.nih.gov/pubmed/28397138. Accessed 14 February 2019.

[3] Ansari SF, Terry C, Cohen-Gadol AA: Surgery for vestibular schwannomas: a systematic review of complications by approach. *Neurosurg. Focus* 33:E14, 2012 Available: http://www.ncbi.nlm.nih.gov/pubmed/22937848. Accessed 14 February 2019.

[4] Chamoun R, MacDonald J, Shelton C, Couldwell WT: Surgical approaches for resection of vestibular schwannomas: translabyrin-

thine, retrosigmoid, and middle fossa approaches. *Neurosurg. Focus* E9, 2012 Available: https://thejns.org/view/journals/neurosurg-focus/33/3/article-pE9.xml. Accessed 14 February 2019.

[5] Da Silva C, da Silva JB, da Silva V: Use of sodium fluorescein in skull base tumors. *Surg. Neurol. Int.* 1:70, 2010 Available: http://www.ncbi.nlm.nih.gov/pubmed/21125008. Accessed 14 February 2019.

[6] DeMonte F, Gidley PW: Hearing preservation surgery for vestibular schwannoma: experience with the middle fossa approach. *Neurosurg. Focus* E10, 2012 Available: https://thejns.org/view/journals/neurosurg-focus/33/3/article-pE10.xml. Accessed 14 February 2019.

[7] Francaviglia N, Iacopino DGD, Costantino G, Villa A, Impallaria P, Meli F, et al. Fluorescein for resection of high-grade gliomas: A safety study control in a single center and review of the literature. *Surg. Neurol. Int.* 8:145, 2017 Available: http://surgicalneurologyint.com/surgicalint-articles/fluorescein-for-resection-of-high-grade-gliomas-a-safety-study-control-in-a-single-center-and-review-of-the-literature/%0Ahttp://www.ncbi.nlm.nih.gov/pubmed/28781922%0Ahttp://www.pubmedcentral.nih.gov/a.

[8] Giammalva G, Iacopino D, Maugeri R: Natura abhorret a vacuo. Future perspectives of autologous fibrin glue. Is it time for reappraisal? *Surg. Neurol. Int.* 8:2017.

[9] Giugno A, Maugeri R, D'Arpa S, Visocchi M, Iacopino DG: Complex reconstructive surgery following removal of extra-intracranial meningiomas, including the use of autologous fibrin glue and a pedicled muscle flap. *Interdiscip. Neurosurg. Adv. Tech. Case Manag.* 1:84-87, 2014.

[10] Grasso G, Meli F, Fodale V, Calapai G, Buemi M, Iacopino DG: Neuroprotective potential of erythropoietin and darbepoetin alfa in an experimental model of sciatic nerve injury. *J. Neurosurg. Spine* 7:645-651, 2007 Available: http://thejns.org/doi/10.3171/SPI-07/12/645.

[11] Graziano F, Certo F, Basile L, Maugeri R, Grasso G, Meccio F, et al. Autologous fibrin sealant (Vivostat®) in the neurosurgical practice:

Part I: Intracranial surgical procedure. *Surg. Neurol. Int*. 6:77, 2015 Available: http://www.ncbi.nlm.nih.gov/pubmed/25984391.

[12] Graziano F, Maugeri R, Basile L, Meccio F, Iacopino D: Aulogous fibrin sealant (Vivostat®) in the neurosurgical practice: Part II: Vertebro-spinal procedures. *Surg. Neurol. Int*. 7:77, 2016 Available: http://surgicalneurologyint.com/surgicalint_articles/aulogous-fibrin-sealant-vivostat-in-the-neurosurgical-practice-part-ii-vertebro-spinal-procedures/.

[13] H. Richard Winn M: Youmans & Winn Neurological Surgery. *Youmans Winn Neurol. Surg*. 2017.

[14] House WF, Shelton C: Middle Fossa Approach for Acoustic Tumor Removal. *Neurosurg. Clin. N. Am.* 19:279-288, 2008 Available: https://linkinghub.elsevier.com/retrieve/pii/S1042368008000107. Accessed 14 February 2019.

[15] Kang WS, Kim SA, Yang CJ, Nam SH, Chung JW: Surgical outcomes of middle fossa approach in intracanalicular vestibular schwannoma. *Acta Otolaryngol*. 137:352-355, 2017 Available: https://www.tandfonline.com/doi/full/10.1080/00016489.2016.1255992. Accessed 14 February 2019.

[16] Kutz JW, Scoresby T, Isaacson B, Mickey BE, Madden CJ, Barnett SL, et al. Hearing Preservation Using the Middle Fossa Approach for the Treatment of Vestibular Schwannoma. *Neurosurgery* 70:334-341, 2012 Available: https://academic.oup.com/neurosurgery/article-lookup/doi/10.1227/NEU.0b013e31823110f1. Accessed 14 February 2019.

[17] La Torre D, Maugeri R, Angileri FF, Pezzino G, Conti A, Cardali SM, et al. Human leukocyte antigen frequency in human high-grade gliomas: a case-control study in Sicily. *Neurosurgery* 64:1082-8; discussion 1088-9, 2009.

[18] Scorpecci A, Massoud M, Giannantonio S, Zangari P, Lucidi D, Martines F, Foligno S, Di Felice G, Minozzi A, Luciani M, Marsella P (2018) Otogenic lateral sinus thrombosis in children: proposal of an experience-based treatment flowchart. *European Archives of Oto-Rhino-Laryngology*, 275 (8), pp. 1971-1977.

[19] Maugeri R, Villa A, Pino M, Imperato A, Giammalva GR, Costantino G, et al. With a little help from my friends: The role of intraoperative fluorescent dyes in the surgical management of high-grade gliomas. *Brain Sci*. 8:2018.

[20] Maugeri R, Basile L, Giugno A, Graziano F, Iacopino DG: Impasse in the management of recurrent basal cell carcinoma of the skull with sagittal sinus erosion. *Interdiscip. Neurosurg*. 2:160-163, 2015 Available: https://www.sciencedirect.com/science/article/pii/S2214751915300086?via%3Dihub. Accessed 17 September 2018.

[21] Maugeri R, Giammalva GR, Graziano F, Iacopino DG: May Autologue Fibrin Glue Alone Enhance Ossification? An Unexpected Spinal Fusion. *World Neurosurg*. 95:611-612, 2016.

[22] Maugeri R, Schiera G, di Liegro CM, Fricano A, Iacopino DG, Di Liegro I: Aquaporins and brain tumors. *Int. J. Mol. Sci*. 17:2016.

[23] Montaser AS, Todeschini AB, Harris MS, Adunka OF, Prevedello DM: Role of Endoscopy in Resection of Intracanalicular Vestibular Schwannoma via Middle Fossa Approach: Technical Nuances. *World Neurosurg*. 120:395-399, 2018 Available: http://www.ncbi.nlm.nih.gov/pubmed/30201576. Accessed 14 February 2019.

[24] Di Stadio A, Dipietro L, Toffano R, Burgio F, De Lucia A, Ippolito V, Garofalo S, Ricci G, Martines F, Trabalzini F, Della Volpe A (2018) Working memory function in children with single side deafness using a bone-anchored hearing implant: A case-control study. *Audiology and Neurotology*, 23 (4), pp. 238-244.

[25] De Stefano A, Kulamarva G, Dispenza F (2012) Malignant paroxysmal positional vertigo. *Auris Nasus Larynx*, 39:378-.

[26] Sameshima T, Fukushima T, McElveen JT, Friedman AH: Critical assessment of operative approaches for hearing preservation in small acoustic neuroma surgery: retrosigmoid vs middle fossa approach. *Neurosurgery* 67:640-4; discussion 644-5, 2010 Available: https://academic.oup.com/neurosurgery/article/67/3/640/2556958. Accessed 14 February 2019.

[27] Scheich M, Ginzkey C, Ehrmann-Müller D, Shehata-Dieler W, Hagen R: Management of CSF leakage after microsurgery for

vestibular schwannoma via the middle cranial fossa approach. *Eur. Arch. Oto-Rhino-Laryngology* 273:2975-2981, 2016 Available: http://link.springer.com/10.1007/s00405-015-3891-3. Accessed 14 February 2019.

[28] Dispenza F, De Stefano A, Costantino C, Rando D, Giglione M, Stagno R, Bennici F (2015) Canal switch and re entry phenomenon in benign paroxysmal positional vertigo: Difference between immediate and delayed occurrence. *Acta otorhinolaryngol. Ital.*, 35: 116-120.

[29] Scheich M, Ginzkey C, Reuter E, Harnisch W, Ehrmann D, Hagen R: Quality of life after microsurgery for vestibular schwannoma via the middle cranial fossa approach. *Eur. Arch. Oto-Rhino-Laryngology* 271:1909-1916, 2014 Available: http://link.springer.com/10.1007/s00405-013-2671-1. Accessed 14 February 2019.

[30] Dispenza F, Battaglia AM, Salvago P, Martines F (2018) Determinants of failure in the reconstruction of the tympanic membrane: A case-control study. *Iranian Journal Otorhinolaryngology*, 30: 341-346.

[31] Tanriover N, Sanus GZ, Ulu MO, Tanriverdi T, Akar Z, Rubino PA, et al. Middle fossa approach: microsurgical anatomy and surgical technique from the neurosurgical perspective. *Surg. Neurol.* 71:586-596, 2009 Available: http://www.ncbi.nlm.nih.gov/pubmed/18617228. Accessed 14 February 2019.

[32] Teschner M, Lang CP, Salcher R, Haumann S, Lenarz T: Impact of Elevation of Temporal Lobe During Middle Fossa Acoustic Neuroma Surgery on Contralateral Speech Discrimination. *Otol. Neurotol.* 36:1720-4, 2015 Available: https://insights.ovid.com/crossref?an=00129492-201512000-00024. Accessed 14 February 2019.

[33] Wang AC, Chinn SB, Than KD, Arts HA, Telian SA, El-Kashlan HK, et al. Durability of hearing preservation after microsurgical treatment of vestibular schwannoma using the middle cranial fossa approach. *J. Neurosurg.* 119:131-8, 2013 Available: http://www.ncbi.nlm.nih.gov/pubmed/23413947. Accessed 14 February 2019.

In: Vestibular Schwannoma ISBN: 978-1-53617-191-4
Editors: Francesco Dispenza et al.

Chapter 10

ENDOSCOPIC APPROACH TO VESTIBULAR SCHWANNOMA

Daniele Marchioni[1], MD
and Davide Soloperto[1,*], MD, PhD
[1]ENT Department, AOUI Verona, Verona University, Verona, Italy

ABSTRACT

Endoscopic approach is an alternative surgical technique developed for the management of VSs limited to the IAC, minimizing intraoperative and postoperative complications.

After several cadaver dissections to better understand the anatomy and to define appropriate instruments for the surgery, some advances were made in exploring the inner ear: from the labyrinth, jugular, and carotid to the IAC, until an appropriate procedure was recorded and ready to be applied clinically.

Improving the experience in endoscopic ear surgery, the most important advantage in performing surgery in these tumors with endoscopic approach was the reduction of postoperative morbility, that was comparable to that of a tympanoplasty rather than an operation of the

* Corresponding Author's Email: davidesolop@gmail.com.

CPA. In conclusion, in the author's opinion, the transcanal surgery, with TTEA and/or ETA technique, can be added in the "decision making" algorhytm for the management of VS.

Surgical approaches to pathology extending into internal auditory canal (IAC), such as vestibular schwannomas (VSs), are widely known and have been extensively recorded.

The retrosigmoid, middle cranial fossa and translabyrinthine approaches are the most commonly used and well-documented approaches in VS surgery [1, 2]. The choice of the right approach depends on factors such as the surgeon's preferences and habits, dimensions and extent of the pathology, the aim regarding hearing preservation, risk to the facial nerve, and postoperative complications [3]. Having the access the internal auditory canal (IAC) and cerebellopontine angle (CPA), all of these approaches require wide external incisions and a variable degree of temporal bone removal. Considering that the goal of this surgery is to eradicate the tumor, preserving facial nerve (FN) function as much as possible, using sufficient exposure to minimize surgical morbidity, an alternative surgical technique was developed for the management of VSs limited to the IAC, minimizing intraoperative and postoperative complications. The first introduction of the endoscopic technique in IAC surgery has been in combination with the retrosigmoid approach after removal of the CPA extension of the neoplasm [4]. The intracanalicular extension was removed under endoscopic control, trying to avoid extensive drilling of the posterior aspect of the petrous bone. After a gradual introduction of the endoscope in middle ear surgery since 1990 in combination with the microscope, gradually it was used in surgery to replace it as the main tool during middle ear operations [5-9]. After several cadaver dissections to better understand the anatomy and to define appropriate instruments for the surgery, some advances were made in exploring the inner ear: from the labyrinth, jugular, and carotid to the IAC, until an appropriate procedure was recorded and ready to be applied clinically (see figure 1).

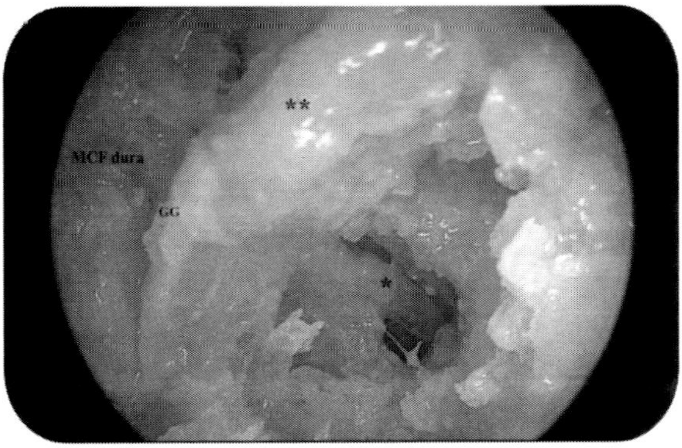

Figure 1. Transcanal endoscopic dissection of the fundus/IAC in a cadaveric specimen (left side). (MCF: middle cranial fossa dura; * intrameatal facial nerve;** tympanic tract of the facial nerve; GG: geniculate ganglion, with greater petrosal nerve course).

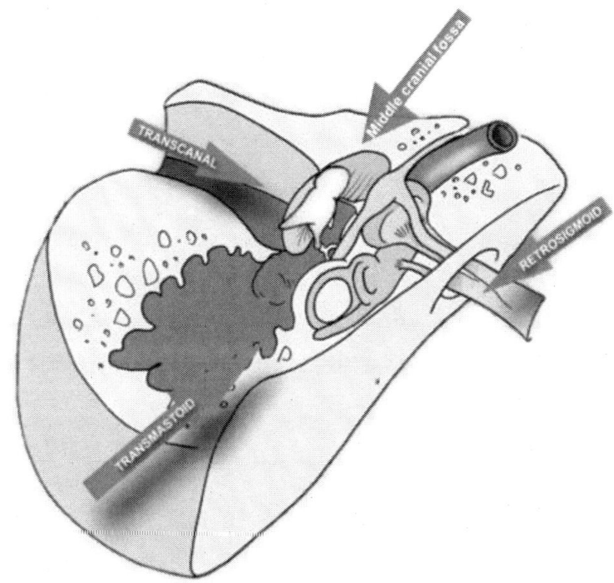

Figure 2. Drawing illustrating all surgical routes for the IAC and CPA.

In 2012, endoscopic access to the lateral skull base through the external auditory canal was realized in a cadaveric study [10] and, in March 2012, for the first time, an exclusive endoscopic approach to the IAC was described and used to remove a VS involving both the IAC and cochlea in a 40 years old patient with hearing loss, tinnitus and vertigo, unresponsive to medical treatment. This approach was called ''transcanal transpromontorial approach'' [11] (see figure 2). The goal of this technique was to reach lesions of the IAC and lateral skull base avoiding craniotomy, brain, middle and posterior fossa manipulations and jugular bulb management, and performing minimally invasive surgery using the external auditory canal, a natural orifice, as direct corridor to the internal auditory canal, in the same fashion as the nasal corridor is used for anterior skull base surgery. In 2017, the first case series of 10 patients with intracanalicular VS who had been treated by an exclusive endoscopic transcanal transpromontorial approach (EETTA) [12]. After this clinical application, this approach was more progressively used in patients with Koos Grade I or II VS, providing high magnification of every structure inside and outside the IAC, including the facial nerve. Improving the experience in endoscopic ear surgery, the most important advantage in performing surgery in these tumors with endoscopic approach was the reduction of postoperative morbility, that was comparable to that of a tympanoplasty rather than an operation of the CPA. The enthusiasm and popularity for this surgery increased and other authors showed their preliminary results with this approach, with a slightly modified EETTA [13], or with some limited case series [14]. The TEA was reported to be very helpful not only for VS limited to the fundus/IAC, but also for the surgical management of intralabirynthic VS, and eight patients affected by an intralabyrinthine schwannoma, with or without extension to the internal auditory canal, were reported to be successfully treated with a transcanal transpromontorial approach [15] (see figure 3, 4, 5, 6, 7, 8).

Bytheway, the indications for the exclusive endoscopic transcanal transpromontorial approach were initially limited to growing VS Koos stage I or II, with class D hearing (AAO-HNS) and whose symptoms does not respond to medical treatment [11, 16].

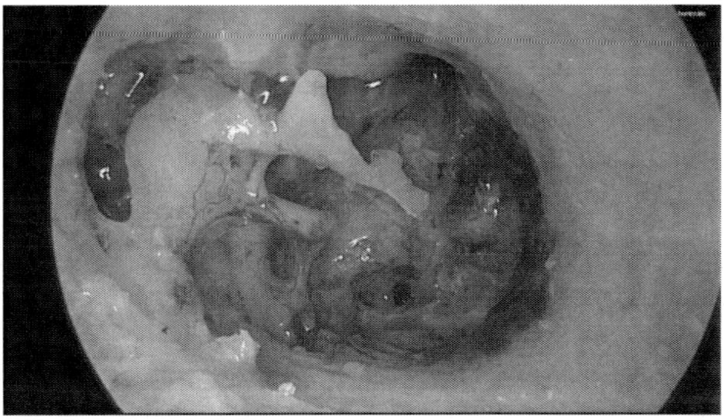

Figure 3. Endoscopic view of right ear. TTEA approach. The skin of the external auditory canal with the tympanic membrane was removed, an atticotomy was performed to expose the ossicular chain.

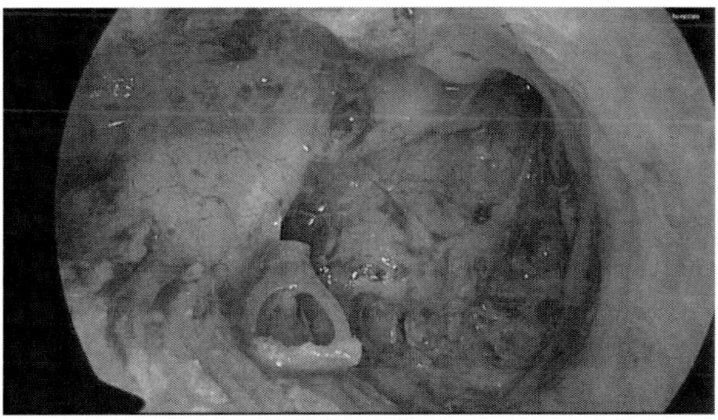

Figure 4. Endoscopic view of right ear. TTEA approach. The ossicular chain was disarticulated and stapes removed, opening the vestibule.

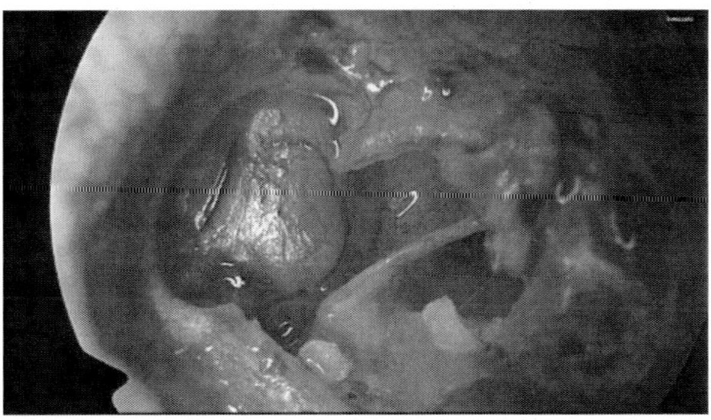

Figure 5. Endoscopic view of right ear. TTEA approach. The neuroma is visible into the vestibule, showing an extension to the funds of the IAC, the cochlea and the lateral semicircular canal (LSC). Note the cochlea completely opened, exposing basal, medium and apical turns.

With the improvement in anatomical and surgical knowledge, this technique was increased adopted also for lesions involving the whole IAC with extension into the CPA (Koos stages II – III). This was possible using the same anatomical landmarks through the external auditory canal enlarging the surgical access using the ETA.

This "enlarged" microscopic two-handed technique permitted improving the surgical window on the CPA, allowing removal of the AN and the management of the vascular structures lying in the CPA. Thus the ETA represented an evolution of the TTEA, being suitable for bigger ANs.

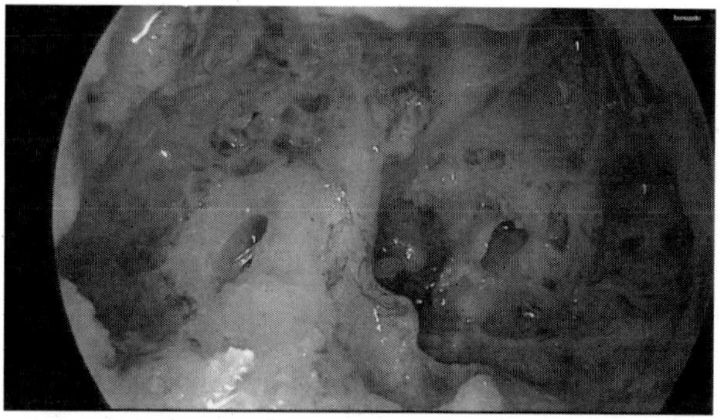

Figure 6. Endoscopic view of right ear. TTEA approach. Note the LSC opened endoscopically, with exposure of the vestibule and cochlea, due to the extension of the tumor requiring this surgical window.

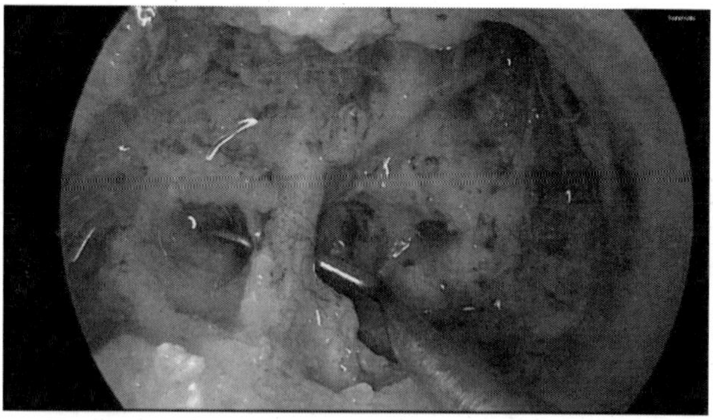

Figure 7. Endoscopic view of right ear. TTEA approach. It's important to underline the course of the tympanic tract of the facial nerve, between the LSC and the pyramidal eminence.

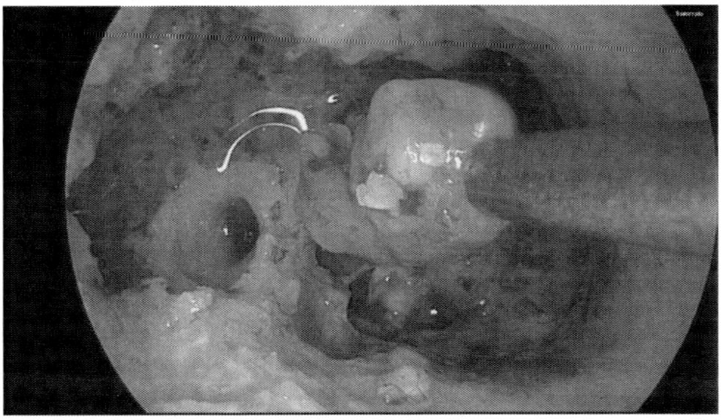

Figure 8. Endoscopic view of right ear. TTEA approach. Tumor removal at the end of the surgery.

Indications were so progressively extended to larger VS, at Koos stages II and III specifically, tumors up to 3cm in size with linear progression into the CPA and with brainstem involvement [17].

Between 2015 and 2017 20 patients affected by Koos stage II and III VS underwent surgery with the ExpTT approach, reporting the best features of the microscopic and endoscopic techniques combined to perform a minimally invasive approach with bimanual dissection, easy control of bleedings, as well as direct identification of anatomic landmarks. This combined technique permits direct access to the IAC and CPA without wide external incisions and extended bone removal, as required by the traditional approaches [18].

The possibility to avoid postoperative intensive care unit recovery is an important advantage in terms of not only a reduction of complications but also economic saving. Bearing in mind that FN function is usually considered to be the best indicator of QoL following VS surgery, the major report of transcanal VS surgery, with TTEA and ETA approach, was reported in 2017. 49 patients who underwent surgery with a totally transcanal exclusive endoscopic approach for Koos stage I – II lesions, or an enlarged transcanal transpromontorial approach for Koos stage II – III tumors, between March 2012 and February 2017 were analyzed (see figure 9,10). Focussing on FN results, overall FN function was perfectly preserved in 95.9% of patients after surgery and results were stable at the last follow-up. Considering the results by surgical approach, FN function was preserved (grade I – II HB) in 100% of ETA, while 90.5% of TTEA had it preserved (grade I – II), but in 9.5% of TTEA cases, it had deteriorated, even if it was not worse than grade III HB, so a normal FN function is present after surgery in 95.9% of patients [19]. These results, if compared with other options ("wait and scan", radiotherapy and traditional microscopic surgeries), are very encouraging. In conclusion, in the author's opinion, the transcanal surgery, with TTEA and/or ETA technique, can be added in the "decision making" algorhytm for the management of VS. It is very promising, since it potentially differs in terms of morbidity from classic microscopic approaches and guarantees radical removal of the pathology, with a possible very low morbidity to the facial nerve, due to direct control and magnification of the entire nerve path thanks to the endoscope.

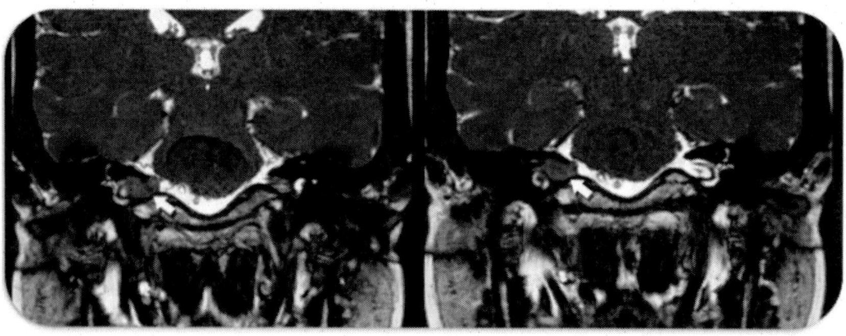

Figure 9. MRI of a Koos stage 1 neuroma on the left side. In these cases a ETTA approach is feasible to reach and remove the tumor.

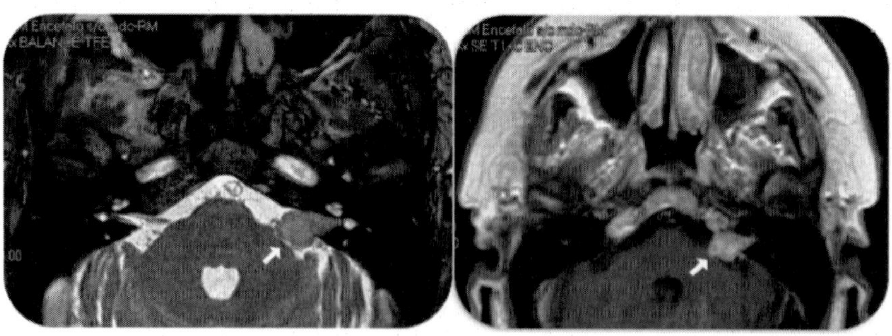

Figure 10. MRI of a Koos stage III neuroma on the right side. In these cases a ETA approach is feasible to reach and remove the tumor.

Actually, to our knowledge hearing preservation is till now not feasible with this approach, but new studies are changing prospective for cochlear preservation and cochlear implantation in the future [20].

REFERENCES

[1] Isaacson, B., Telian, S. A., El-Kashlan, H. K. Facial nerve outcomes in middle cranial fossa vs translabyrinthine approaches. *Otolaryngol. Head Neck Surg.*, 2005; 133:906 - 10.

[2] Cushing, H. *Tumors of the Nervus Acousticus and the Syndrome of the Cerebellopontine Angle*. Philadelphia, PA: WB Saunders; 1917.

[3] Bennett, M., Haynes, D. S. Surgical approaches and complications in the removal of vestibular schwannomas. *Otolaryngol. Clin. North Am.,* 2007; 40:589 - 609.

[4] Magnan, J., Chays, A., Lepetre, C., Pencroffi, E., Locatelli, P. Surgical perspectives of endoscopy of the cerebellopontine angle. *Am. J. Otol.,* 1994; 15:366 - 370.

[5] Tarabichi, M. Endoscopic management of limited attic cholesteatoma. *Laryngoscope,* 2004; 114:1157 - 1162.

[6] Marchioni, D., Soloperto, D., Rubini, A., Nogueira, J. F., Badr-El-Dine, M., Presutti, L. Endoscopic Facial Nerve Surgery. *Otolaryngol. Clin. North Am.,* 2016 Oct.; 49(5):1173 - 87. doi: 10.1016/j.otc.2016.05.006. Epub 2016 Jul 26. Review.

[7] Marchioni, D., Soloperto, D., Colleselli, E., Tatti, M. F., Patel, N., Jufas, N. Round window chamber and fustis: endoscopic anatomy and surgical implications. *Surg. Radiol. Anat.,* 2016 Nov.; 38(9): 1013 - 1019. Epub 2016 Mar. 14.

[8] Marchioni, D., Soloperto, D., Rubini, A., Villari, D., Genovese, E., Artioli, F., Presutti, L. Endoscopic exclusive transcanal approach to the tympanic cavity cholesteatoma in pediatric patients: our experience. *Int. J. Pediatr. Otorhinolaryngol.,* 2015 Mar.; 79(3):316 - 22. doi: 10.1016/j.ijporl.2014.12.008. Epub 2015 Jan 7.

[9] Presutti, L., Marchioni, D., Mattioli, F., Villari, D., Alicandri-Ciufelli, M. Endoscopic management of acquired cholesteatoma: our experience. *J. Otolar- yngol. Head Neck Surg.,* 2008; 37:481 - 487.

[10] Marchioni, D., Alicandri-Ciufelli, M., Rubini, A., Presutti, L. Endoscopic transcanal corridors to the lateral skull base: Initial experi- ences. *Laryngoscope,* 2015; 125 (suppl. 5):S1 3.

[11] Presutti, L., Alicandri-Ciufelli, M., Cigarini, E., Marchioni, D. Cochlear schwannoma removed through the external auditory canal by a transcanal exclusive endoscopic technique. *Laryngoscope,* 2013; 123:2862 - 7.

[12] Marchioni, D., Alicandri-Ciufelli, M., Rubini, A., Masotto, B., Pavesi, G., Presutti, L. Exclusive endoscopic transcanal trans-promontorial approach: a new perspective for internal auditory canal vestibular schwannoma treatment. *J. Neurosurg.,* 2017 Jan.; 126(1):98 - 105. Doi 10.3171/2015.11.JNS15952. Epub 2016 Mar. 11.

[13] Moon, I. S., Cha, D., Nam, S. I., Lee, H. J., Choi, J. Y. The Feasibility of a Modified Exclusive Endoscopic Transcanal Transpromontorial Approach for Vestibular Schwannomas. *Neurol. Surg. B Skull Base,* 2019 Feb.; 80(1):82 - 87. doi: 10.1055/s-0038-1667061. Epub 2018 Jul. 30.

[14] Wick, C. C., Arnaoutakis, D., Barnett, S. L., Rivas, A., Isaacson, B. Endoscopic Transcanal Transpromontorial Approach for Vestibular Schwannoma Resection: A Case Series. *Otol. Neurotol.,* 2017 Dec.; 38 (10):e490 - e494.

[15] Marchioni, D., De Rossi, S., Soloperto, D., Presutti, L., Sacchetto, L., Rubini, A. Intralabyrinthine schwannomas: a new surgical treatment. *Eur. Arch. Otorhinolaryngol.,* 2018 May; 275(5):1095 - 1102. doi: 10.1007/s00405-018-4937-0. Epub 2018 Mar 20.

[16] Marchioni, D., Alicandri-Ciufelli, M., Rubini, A. et al. Exclusive endoscopic transcanal transpromontorial approach: a new perspective for internal auditory canal vestibular schwannoma treatment. *J. Neurosurg.,* 2017; 126:98 - 105.

[17] Marchioni, D., Carner, M., Soloperto, D., Bianconi, L., Sacchetto, A., Sacchetto, L., Masotto, B., Presutti, L. Expanded Transcanal Transpromontorial Approach: A Novel Surgical Technique for Cerebellopontine Angle Vestibular Schwannoma Removal. *Otolaryngol. Head Neck Surg.,* 2018 Apr.; 158(4):710 - 715. Epub 2018 Feb. 6.

[18] Ansari, S. F., Terry, C., Cohen-Gadol, A. A. Surgery for vestibular schwannomas: a systematic review of complications by approach. *Neurosurg. Focus,* 2012; 33:E14.

[19] Marchioni, D., Soloperto, D., Masotto, B., Fabbris, C., De Rossi, S., Villari, D., Presutti, L. Transcanal Transpromontorial Acoustic Neuroma Surgery: Results and Facial Nerve Outcomes. *Otol. Neurotol.,* 2018 Feb.; 39(2):242 - 249.

[20] Marchioni, D., Veronese, S., Carner, M., Sacchetto, A., Sacchetto, L., Masotto, B., Bianconi, L. Hearing Restoration During Vestibular Schwannoma Surgery With Transcanal Approach: Anatomical and Functional Preliminary Report. *Neurotol.,* 2018 Dec.; 39(10):1304 - 1310.

In: Vestibular Schwannoma ISBN: 978-1-53617-191-4
Editors: Francesco Dispenza et al.

Chapter 11

RADIOTHERAPY FOR VESTIBULAR SCHWANNOMA

***Gianluca Mortellaro*[1,*], *Giuseppe Ferrera*[1], *Francesco Cuccia*[2] and *Filippo Alongi*[3,4]**
[1]Radiation Oncology Unit, ARNAS Ospedale Civico Di Cristina Benfratelli, Palermo, Italy
[2]Radiation Oncology School, University of Palermo, Palermo, Italy
[3]Advanced Radiation Oncology Department, IRCCS, Ospedale Sacro Cuore Don Calabria, Negrar, Verona, Italy
[4]University of Brescia, Brescia Italy

ABSTRACT

The role of radiotherapy for the treatment of VS has been established since the first Gamma-knife radiosurgery experiences took place in 1969. The constant progress of technology allowed the development of more accurate systems able to ensure the safe irradiation of deep located lesions, inaccessible for neurosurgery, with a reduced risk of radiation-related damages. This led to consider the use of radiation therapy an iso-

* Corresponding Author's Email: gianlucamortellaro@virgilio.it.

effective alternative to surgery, with a smaller impact on neurological sequelae. Nowadays, radiotherapy for VS can be delivered with stereotactic radiosurgery, conventional fractionation, hypofractionation and particle therapy.

INTRODUCTION

Radiotherapy is a consolidated option for the treatment of tumors that uses high doses of high-energy ionizing radiations to kill cancer cells by damaging their *DNA*. Cells whose DNA is damaged beyond repair stop dividing, growing or die. This allows to gain excellent tumor control rates and, consequently, increased survival outcomes. External beam radiation therapy (EBRT) is delivered by linear accelerators (LINACs). In some cases of intracranial masses located in critical sites hardly suitable for surgery, radiotherapy can be proposed as an attractive choice for the treatment of either malignant or benign neoplasms, including vestibular Schwannoma (VS). For these peculiar targets, the goal for successful treatment is represented by the delivery of a high dose of radiations to the tumor site, minimizing the exposure of the nearby healthy structures, whether using conventional fractionation (1.8–2 Gy per fraction), hypofractionation (>2 Gy per fraction) or radiosurgery.

Current therapeutic options for VS include observation, microsurgery, radiotherapy. The role of radiotherapy for the treatment of VS has been established since the first Gamma-knife radiosurgery experiences took place in 1969 [1]. The constant progress of technology allowed the development of more accurate systems able to ensure the safe irradiation of deep located lesions, inaccessible for neurosurgery, with a reduced risk of radiation-related damages. This led to consider the use of radiation therapy an iso-effective alternative to surgery, with a smaller impact on neurological sequelae [2]. Nowadays, radiotherapy for VS can be delivered with stereotactic radiosurgery, conventional fractionation, hypo-fractionation and particle therapy.

TECIINICAL ASPECTS OF STEREOTACTIC RADIOSURGERY AND MODERN RADIOTHERAPY

The term "stereotactic radiosurgery" was introduced in 1951, when Lars Leksell mentioned a theoretical method for "the non-invasive destruction of intracranial lesions." After the introduction of the first stereotactic frame, few years later, he developed the definitive concept of radiosurgery [3, 4]. Thanks to the capability to localize, with a high grade of accuracy, a target in three-dimensional space, Leksell affirmed that narrow beams of radiation intersecting at a common point could allow clinicians to concentrate high doses of radiation to a target volume inside the brain [5]. With this specific method, tumors located deeply within the brain tissue or at the base of the skull could be irradiated with minimal damage to surrounding healthy critical structures. Further researches culminated in the development of the Gamma knife Unit [6]. In the late 1980s, at the University of Florida, a team of neurosurgeons, radiation physicists and engineers developed the first LINAC-based radiosurgery delivery system [7]. After that, using LINAC-based system at the University of Florida, more than 2000 patients have been treated with radiosurgery. From the beginning of the 1990s, various other LINAC-based radiosurgery systems are available in clinical practice and, to date, it is the most commonly adopted approach for SRS delivery worldwide.

From technical point of view, SRS is a radiation technique capable to deliver, in a single session, an extremely high dose of ionizing radiation toward an intracranial target; the tumor is usually identified using stereotactic parameters on imaging, performed before and during the SRS procedure. The radiation tolerability of normal tissue is dependent on irradiated volume, and SRS exploits this concept delivering high conformal doses to small targets. With stereotactic techniques, the expected sequelae depending on radiation dose delivered to healthy surrounding tissues are limited, minimizing or eliminating the margins of the critical structures close to the planning treatment volume, usually compromised with conventional radiotherapy techniques. The most commonly available SRS systems are based on high-energy X-rays generated from a clinical LINAC. The intersection of the axis of rotation of the gantry and the treatment couch and the central axis of the photon beam is a point defined as the LINAC isocenter. Planning Target Volumes could be treated using single or multiple isocenter plans. Classic stereotactic LINAC technology uses circular collimators of different diameters from 3-5mm to 50 mm. Intensity Modulated Radiation techniques (IMRT) can also be utilized as an SRS treatment delivery method, mainly to improve accuracy when compared with conventional stereotactic delivery systems. IMRT treatment should be carefully performed using three-dimensional images of the patient in conjunction with complex dose calculation algorithms to create the dose intensity pattern for the best conformity to the treatment volume shape. Usually, various combinations of several intensity-modulated fields with different beam directions generate a custom tailored radiation dose. The result is that dose distribution optimized target coverage, while better sparing adjacent healthy tissues exposed to higher radiation doses.

Moreover, specific machines designed for SRS, or stereotactic body radiotherapy have been clinically implemented, recently. Cyberknife technology is based on a robotic arm that allows the delivery of the radiation dose using hundreds of non-isocentric and non-coplanar beams gaining highly conformal dose distributions. Stereotactic targeting is more accurate and precise due to the combination of real-time orthogonal x-ray imaging with a sophisticated image recognition platform for the automatic tracking of bony structures or implanted fiducials, overcoming the need of rigid devices for fixation.

Treatment positioning is another crucial element for precision SRS delivery: the head of the patient is aligned to the LINAC beam and immobilized with a personalized thermoplastic mask. In modern LINAC systems dedicated to SRS, a robotic couch is frequently provided, to further reduce uncertainties of patient positioning when compared to planned parameters, and volumetric Image Guidance systems (IGRT) are adopted to minimize set-up error corrections before and after treatment session. IGRT is available on LINACs as various kinds of integrated imaging systems on board: very high quality of images, as well as KV cone beam CT or MV CT and/or electronic portal images, are commonly equipped for SRS and precise treatments on LINACs. Due to the capability to correct set up uncertainties with a very high resolution quality of images, more comfortable frameless immobilization devices are even more used for SRS patients when combined with IMRT-IGRT delivery.

RADIOSURGERY CLINICAL EXPERIENCES

Since observation was considered the first choice for patients with small tumors and minimal burden of symptoms, at first, SRS was indicated for elderly patients, medically inoperable or in case of bilateral disease, and as a salvage option for recurrence after surgery. The first literature experiences concerning the use of SRS for VS were similar in regard to the adoption of high dose schedules, between 14 and 25 Gy delivered in a single fraction, resulting in excellent local control rates (90-100%). Nevertheless, a relative higher incidence of adverse events when compared to the post-surgery complications rates was reported. [8] Particularly, Suh et al. [9] in their series of 29 patients treated with 16 Gy SRS observed a hearing dysfunction in 74% of cases, while new or worsening trigeminal and facial neuropathies were observed in 15% and 32%, respectively. Similarly, Foote et al. [10], in their series of 36 VS treated with a marginal dose of 16-20 Gy, recorded 2-year actuarial rates of hearing preservation of 41.7%, while 2-years incidence rate of facial and/or trigeminal nerve deficits was 81.7%. In a larger cohort of 162 Gamma-knife patients, Kondziolka et al [11], after five years of follow-up, collected similar results, with excellent 98% local control rates, while hearing loss was observed in 49% of cases, facial nerve neuropathy in 21% and trigeminal dysfunction in 27%. In light of the high rates of tumor control, subsequent studies evaluated the possibility of dose de-escalation, paying more attention to functional outcomes and hearing, trigeminal and facial nerve preservation.

One of the largest data series collected about the prescription of lower doses of 12-13 Gy SRS has been reported by the University of Pittsburgh

[12]: in their series of 313 patients with VS, a 7-years actuarial tumor control rate of 98.6% was reported, while hearing, facial and trigeminal nerve preservation rates were respectively 78.6%, 100% and 96.6%. Particularly for trigeminal function, the authors observed a higher risk of neuropathy in patients with a larger tumor volume (p = 0.038). Similarly, dose de-escalation confirmed analogous results in other published papers reinforcing the adoption of the 11-13 Gy SRS prescription, subsequently evaluated in larger cohorts [13-16].

In 2013, Hasegawa et al. [17] published data about 440 patients treated with Gamma-knife for a median dose of 12.8 Gy in a single fraction. This series collects the longest median follow-up of 12.5 years reporting 5- and 10-years rates of tumor control of 93% and 92%, while hearing preservation rates were 43% at 5 years, and 34% at 8 years.

In a larger series of 523 patients treated with median 13 Gy Gamma-knife SRS, Boari et al. [18] collected local control rates of 97.1%, with overall functional hearing preservation of 49%, reporting only late temporary worsening of symptoms already existing at the baseline.

Furthermore, interesting data come from the prospective study by Breivik et al. [19], in a cohort of 237 patients with VS receiving SRS or observation: no significant difference in terms of hearing dysfunction between the two options were recorded, detecting hearing loss in 64% of the radiosurgery arm vs 76% in the observation group. Concerning clinical outcomes, a statistically significant tumor downsizing was reported in the SRS sample.

These results lead to the adoption of the currently widespread dose prescription of 11-13 Gy in a single fraction. The favorable combination of lower prescription doses and refined radiotherapy techniques allowed to gain remarkable results both in terms of tumor control and functional preservation, making SRS an attractive and non-invasive alternative to microsurgery; two meta-analyses [20, 21] reported better functional outcomes in the SRS cohorts, and similar tumor control rates between radiotherapy and surgical patients. Recently, a Cochrane review [22] of randomized trials stated that current evidence is not sufficient to prefer micro- or radiosurgery for VS treatment. However, six prospective studies

[21, 23-27] of comparison between surgery and SRS recorded similar effectiveness between the two approaches, with a significant superiority of SRS in terms of neurological late sequelae. A subsequent systematic review of patients, included in these series who were eligible for both Gamma-knife or microsurgery, reported better outcomes in the radiosurgery cohort [28].

Considering the previously discusses capability of LINACs in order to deliver a radiosurgery treatment, achieving a more accurate shape of the target, with homogeneous dose distributions, most of the recent experiences used LINAC-Based SRS techniques. Puataweepong et al. [29] reported the results of a series of 39 patients treated with LINAC-based SRS for small tumors (≤3 cm) collecting 5-years local control and hearing preservation rates of 95% and 75%, respectively. Similar results were also reported by Badakhsi et al. [30] and Ellenbogen et al. [31].

In the last years, several studies [32, 33] have investigated the need of dose constraints for nearby normal structures, particularly for inner ear components, in the effort to provide effective treatment with minimal impact on auditory function. Jacob et al. [34] evaluated long term outcomes of SRS in a cohort of 105 patients focusing on a dosimetric analysis with the aim to identify a threshold dose for the maximum dose of the cochlea. The authors recommend a <5 Gy mean dose, as they observed a significant association between baseline hearing function and marginal dose and mean cochlear dose, but at the same time, they underline the potential risk to under-dose the tumor to achieve a better cochlear sparing. More recently, van Linge et al. [35] evaluated the outcomes of 67 patients treated with LINAC-based SRS and 63 patients treated with fractionated stereotactic radiotherapy, observing that multivariate Cox and linear regression showed a statistically significant association between V90 cochlear EQD2 (i.e., Equivalent Dose in 2 Gy fractions) dose and hearing loss, suggesting that more efforts on reducing V90 may translate in a benefit for the acoustic nerve preservation.

Conventional Fractionation Clinical Experiences

The use of fractionated stereotactic treatments (FSRT) using conventional fractionation (1.8-2 Gy/die) represented a potential option for larger tumors offering the possibility to deliver lower daily doses gaining a better organs' at risk (OARs) sparing, without compromising local control outcomes. The radiobiological rationale of conventionally fractionated schedules lies on the chance of targeting all the tumor cells in the sensitive cell cycle phases, despite VS is a benign slow-growing tumor, with a low α/ß ratio, hence with limited benefits offered by fractionation. Thus, the choice of fractionated schedules seems more appropriate for larger tumors, with irregular shapes and volumes, in the effort to deliver a more conservative treatment in terms of functional outcomes. Conventional treatments are mainly delivered using LINACs, machines able to focus shaped beams of high energy X-rays to a stereotactically located target using collimators to design a dynamic configuration of the irradiation field. To date, total doses >45 Gy using daily 1.8-2 Gy fractions offer similar local control rates to SRS approach [36]. On the other side, compared to radiosurgery, conventionally fractionated schedules impact favorably on the incidence of adverse events, even if some authors hypothesize that long-lasting treatments seem only to delay the onset of late neurological effects rather than decrease their incidence [37]. Current literature is lacking a randomized trial of comparison between SRS and FSRT, with most of the evidence deriving from retrospective studies concluding that the two approaches are equivalent in terms of efficacy and safety [38-40].

A retrospective cohort of 93 patients who underwent 52.5 Gy in 25 fractions schedules reported a 92% overall control rate with a 15 years follow-up period [41] Also, 7% of cases noticed hearing damage, 1% trigeminal dysfunction, 1% facial nerve palsy, 1% brainstem necrosis and 4% developed radiation-induced hydrocephalus. Litre et al. [42] collected data about a series of 158 VS treated with 50.4 Gy using 1.8 Gy per fraction, with 5-years local control rates of 97.5% reporting rates of facial and trigeminal dysfunction in 2.5% and 3.2% of cases, respectively. New onset or worsening tinnitus was described in 2.1%.

Compared to the abovementioned series, Champ et al. [43] reported the outcomes of a cohort of 154 patients treated with a lower total dose of 46.8 Gy in 26 fractions observing 5-years tumor control rate of 93%, and, notably, better hearing preservation rates at 3 and 5 years of 66% and 54% respectively. The favorable results of this series both in terms of clinical and functional outcomes suggest the possibility to evaluate dose de-escalation also in the conventional fractionation setting.

SCHEDULES OF RADIATION HYPOFRACTIONATION

Schedules of hypofractionation (>2 Gy per fraction) have been evaluated for the treatment of VS, despite their potential role is still investigational. Similarly to conventional fractionate approach used for FSRT, the goal of >2 Gy/fx schedules is to reduce the incidence of hearing and neurological late adverse events offering at the same time a shorter overall treatment time that may favorably impact on patient's compliance. First experiences reported different prescriptions, also based on tumor size. Williams et al. [44] reported the outcomes of 150 patients who were treated respectively with 25 Gy in 5 fractions for tumors smaller than 3 cm, and 30 Gy in 10 fractions for larger tumors. As the majority of cases underwent the 5 fractions schedule, after 1 year, the hearing function was maintained in 70% of patients. Similarly, Meijer et al. [45] reported a series of 80 patients treated with two different schedules: 20 Gy in 4 fractions and 25 Gy in 5 fractions, with 5-years local control and facial nerve preservation rates of 94 and 96%, respectively. For both these series, the use of less conformal than current radiosurgery techniques must be taken into account for the evaluation of these results.

In the last years, the worldwide spread of the robotic guided radiotherapy (Cyberknife, Accuray, US) led to the growth of several literature single center experiences for the treatment of VS [46]. In 2005, Chang et al. [47] collected data about 61 patients treated with Cyberknife for VS for total doses of 18 or 21 Gy using three 6- or 7-Gy fractions: with a mean follow-up of 48 months they observed tumor control and hearing preservation rates of 98% and 90%, respectively.

More recently, two series also investigated the use of Cyberknife for the hypofractionated treatment of VS. Hansasuta et al. [48] reported the results of one of the largest series about hypofractionation for VS at the Stanford University Medical Centre, using an 18 Gy in 3 fractions schedule for 383 patients. The authors observed 3 and 5-years tumor control rates of 99% and 96%, with trigeminal dysfunction detected in only 2% of cases, and collecting a hearing preservation rate of 76%; therefore, smaller tumors were found to be statistically associated with a higher hearing preservation rate ($p = 0.001$). The same schedule was investigated in a retrospective study of 117 patients reporting a 99.1% tumor control rate and a hearing preservation rate of 80%, with a median follow-up of 64 months [49]. Also in this series, larger tumors were significantly associated with a higher probability of hearing damage.

PARTICLE THERAPY

Similarly to other tumors of the skull base, also for VS, proton therapy theoretically represents an attractive therapeutic option. Given the almost equivalent radiobiological effect of protons and photons, the peculiar dose distribution of protons, with a rapid dose fall-off after the Bragg peak, allows to better spare the surrounding healthy tissues, maintaining the same efficacy in terms of tumor control. Several data in the literature are available about the use of protons for VS, investigating either SRS, FSRT or hypofractionation [50].

Weber et al. [51] reported data about 88 cases of VS treated with proton-based SRS, collecting, with a median follow-up of 38 months, actuarial 2 and 5-years local control rates of 95.3% and 93.6%, respectively. Concerning functional outcomes, 5-years trigeminal and facial preservation rates were 89% and 91%, hearing preservation rate was

24% in patients with pre-treatment normal hearing function. Hydrocephalus requiring shunt was observed in 3.4%.

Conventional fractionated proton beam therapy was investigated by Bush et al. [52] in a series of 31 VS treated with a total dose of 60 cobalt Gray equivalent (CgyE) delivered in 30-33 fractions. With a mean follow-up of 34 months, the authors observed no local or distant progression on magnetic resonance imaging. Among 13 patients who were assessed for hearing function in the pre-treatment setting, a useful hearing was maintained in 31% of cases, no facial or trigeminal injuries were recorded.

Vernimmen et al. [53] evaluated the use of hypofractionation with protons, in their series of 51 one cases treated with a total dose of 26 CgyE delivered in 3 fractions. After a mean follow-up of 60 months, 5-years local control was 98%, hearing function preservation rate was 42%, trigeminal and facial nerve preservation rates were respectively 93% and 90.5%.

CONCLUSION

Although many data have been published and analyzed on the use of radiotherapy in its multiple forms (SRS, FSRT, Hypofractionated, protons), no consensus on the subject of VS has yet been reached in details. The debate mainly continues whether surgery or SRS is better for this kind of patients. SRS has progressively achieved an important role in the management of VS, and LINAC-based SRS availability in most radiation therapy departments has widened the possibility of access to brain radiosurgery worldwide. Retrospective studies and several randomized trials have shown the benefits of SRS and the relative risks. Undoubted, compared to surgery for SV, radiosurgery avoids the interventional risks of hemorrhage, infection, and tumor seeding, requiring minimal or no hospitalization, reducing the risks and costs of surgical therapy. Thus, LINAC-based SRS or dedicated machines for SRS, including Gamma-knife and Cyberknife, represent a non-invasive, safe and effective treatment option for SV.

References

[1] Leksell L. A note on the treatment of acoustic tumours. *Acta Chir Scand.* 1971;137(8):763-5.

[2] Dispenza F, DE Stefano A, Costantino C, Rando D, Giglione M, Stagno R, Bonnici E. *Canal swich and re-entry phenomenon in benign paroxysmal positional vertigo: difference between immediate and delayed occurrence.* Acta otorhinolaryngologica Italica: organo ufficiale della Societa italiana di otorinolaringologia e chirurgia cervico-facciale [*Canal switch and re-entry phenomenon in benign paroxysmal positional vertigo: difference between immediate and delayed occurrence. Acta otorhinolary-ngologica Italica: official organ of the Italian Society of Otolaryngology and cervico-facial surgery*], 2015; 35(2), 116-20.

[3] Leksell L. The stereotaxic method and radiosurgery of the brain. *Acta Chir Scand.* 1951 Dec 13;102(4):316-9.

[4] Leksell L, Lindquist C, Adler JR, Leksell D, Jernberg B, Steiner L. A new fixation device for the Leksell stereotaxic system. Technical note. *J Neurosurg.* 1987 Apr;66(4):626-9.

[5] Leksell L. Stereotactic radiosurgery. *J Neurol Neurosurg Psychiatry.* 1983 Sep; 46(9):797-803.

[6] Dinka D, Nyce JM, Timpka T. Gamma Knife surgery: safety and the identity of users. *Technol Health Care.* 2005;13(6):485-95.

[7] Friedman WA, Bova FJ. The University of Florida radiosurgery system. *Surg Neurol.* 1989 Nov;32(5):334-42.

[8] Dispenza F, Battaglia AM, Salvago P, Martines F. Determinants of Failure in the Reconstruction of the Tympanic Membrane: A Case-Control Study. *Iran J Otorhinolaryngol.* 2018;30(101):341-346.

[9] Suh JH, Barnett GH, Sohn JW, Kupelian PA, Cohen BH. Results of linear accelerator-based stereotactic radiosurgery for recurrent and newly diagnosed acoustic neuromas. *Int J Cancer.* 2000 Jun 20;90(3):145-51.

[10] Foote RL, Coffey RJ, Swanson JW, Harner SG, Beatty CW, Kline RW, Stevens LN, Hu TC. Stereotactic radiosurgery using the gamma

knife for acoustic neuromas. *Int J Radiat Oncol Biol Phys*. 1995 Jul 15;32(4):1153-60.

[11] Kondziolka D, Lunsford LD, McLaughlin MR, Flickinger JC. Long-term outcomes after radiosurgery for acoustic neuromas. *N Engl J Med*. 1998 Nov 12;339(20):1426-33.

[12] Flickinger JC, Kondziolka D, Niranjan A, Maitz A, Voynov G, Lunsford LD. Acoustic neuroma radiosurgery with marginal tumor doses of 12 to 13 Gy. *Int J Radiat Oncol Biol Phys*. 2004 Sep 1;60(1):225-30.

[13] Iwai Y, Yamanaka K, Shiotani M, Uyama T. Radiosurgery for acoustic neuromas: results of low-dose treatment. *Neurosurgery*. 2003 Aug;53(2):282-87; discussion 287-8.

[14] Muacevic A, Jess-Hempen A, Tonn JC, Wowra B. Results of Outpatient Gamma Knife Radiosurgery for Primary Therapy of Acoustic Neuromas. In: Wowra B, Muacevic A, Tonn JC (eds) Gamma Knife Radiosurgery. *Acta Neurochirurgica Supplements,* 2004 vol 91. Springer, Vienna.

[15] Paek SH, Chung HT, Jeong SS, Park CK, Kim CY, Kim JE, Kim DG, Jung HW. Hearing preservation after gamma knife stereotactic radiosurgery of vestibular schwannoma. *Cancer*. 2005 Aug 1;104(3):580-90.

[16] Rowe J. G., Radatz M. W., Walton L., Hampshire A., Seaman S., Kemeny A. A. Gamma knife stereotactic radiosurgery for unilateral acoustic neuromas. *J Neurol Neurosurg Psychiatry*. 2003 Nov;74(11):1536-42.

[17] Hasegawa T., Kida Y., Kato T., Iizuka H., Kuramitsu S., Yamamoto T. Long-term safety and efficacy of stereotactic radiosurgery for vestibular schwannomas: evaluation of 440 patients more than 10 years after treatment with Gamma Knife surgery. *J Neurosurg*. 2013 Mar; 118(3):557-65.

[18] Scorpecci, A., Massoud, M., Giannantonio, S., Zangari, P., Lucidi, D., Martines, F., Foligno, S., Di Felice, G., Minozzi, A., Luciani, M., Marsella, P. (2018) Otogenic lateral sinus thrombosis in children:

proposal of an experience-based treatment flowchart. *European Archives of Oto-Rhino-Laryngology*, 275 (8), pp. 1971-1977.

[19] Di Stadio, A., Dipietro, L., Toffano, R., Burgio, F., De Lucia, A., Ippolito, V., Garofalo, S., Ricci, G., Martines, F., Trabalzini, F., Della Volpe, A. (2018) Working memory function in children with single side deafness using a bone-anchored hearing implant: A case-control study. *Audiology and Neurotology,* 23 (4), pp. 238-244.

[20] Maniakas A, Saliba I. Microsurgery versus stereotactic radiation for small vestibular schwannomas: a meta-analysis of patients with more than 5 years' follow-up. *Otol Neurotol*. 2012 Dec;33(9):1611-20.

[21] Karpinos M, Teh BS, Zeck O, Carpenter LS, Phan C, Mai WY, Lu HH, Chiu JK, Butler EB, Gormley WB, Woo SY. Treatment of acoustic neuroma: stereotactic radiosurgery vs. microsurgery. *Int J Radiat Oncol Biol Phys*. 2002 Dec 1;54(5):1410-21.

[22] Muzevic D, Legcevic J, Splavski B, Cayé-Thomasen P. Stereotactic radiotherapy for vestibular schwannoma. *Cochrane Database Syst Rev*. 2014 Dec 16;(12):CD009897.

[23] Myrseth E, Møller P, Pedersen PH, Vassbotn FS, Wentzel-Larsen T, Lund-Johansen M. Vestibular schwannomas: clinical results and quality of life after microsurgery or gamma knife radiosurgery. *Neurosurgery*. 2005 May;56(5):927-35; discussion 927-35.

[24] Myrseth E, Møller P, Pedersen PH, Lund-Johansen M. Vestibular schwannoma: surgery or gamma knife radiosurgery? A prospective, nonrandomized study. *Neurosurgery*. 2009 Apr;64(4):654-61; discussion 661-3.

[25] Pollock B. E., Lunsford L. D., Kondziolka D., Flickinger J. C., Bissonette D. J., Kelsey S. F., Jannetta P. J. Outcome analysis of acoustic neuroma management: a comparison of microsurgery and stereotactic radiosurgery. Neurosurgery. 1995 Jan; 36(1):215-24; discussion 224-9. *Erratum in: Neurosurgery* 1995 Feb; 36(2):427.

[26] Pollock, B. E., Driscoll, C. L., Foote, R. L., Link, M. J., Gorman, D. A., Bauch, C. D., Mandrekar, J. N., Krecke, K. N., Johnson, C. H. Patient outcomes after vestibular schwannoma management: a

prospective comparison of microsurgical resection and stereotactic radiosurgery. *Neurosurgery*. 2006 Jul;59(1):77-85; discussion 77-85.

[27] Régis J., Tamura M., Delsanti C., Roche P. H., Pellet W., Thomassin J. M. Hearing preservation in patients with unilateral vestibular schwannoma after gamma knife surgery. *Prog Neurol Surg*. 2008;21:142-51.

[28] De Stefano A., Kulamarva G, Dispenza F. (2012) Malignant paroxysmal positional vertigo. *Auris Nasus Larynx*, 39:378-382

[29] Puataweepong, P., Dhanachai, M., Dangprasert, S., Narkwong, L., Sitathanee, C., Sawangsilpa, T., Janwityanujit, T., Yongvithisatid, P. Linac-based stereotactic radiosurgery and fractionated stereotactic radiotherapy for vestibular schwannomas: comparative observations of 139 patients treated at a single institution. *J Radiat Res*. 2014 Mar 1;55(2):351-8.

[30] Badakhshi, H., Graf R., Böhmer, D., Synowitz, M., Wiener, E., Budach, V. Results for local control and functional outcome after linac-based image-guided stereotactic radiosurgery in 190 patients with vestibular schwannoma. *J Radiat Res*. 2014 Mar 1;55(2):288-92.

[31] Ellenbogen JR, Waqar M, Kinshuck AJ, Jenkinson MD, Lesser TH, Husband D, Javadpour M. Linear accelerator radiosurgery for vestibular schwannomas: Results of medium-term follow-up. *Br J Neurosurg*. 2015;29(5):678-84.

[32] Morrison D. Management of patients with acoustic neuromas: a Markov decision analysis. Laryngoscope. 2010 Apr;120(4):783-90.

[33] Mazzoni A, Krengli M. Historical development of the treatment of skull base tumours. *Rep Pract Oncol Radiother*. 2016 Jul-Aug;21(4):319-24.

[34] Jacob JT, Carlson ML, Schiefer TK, Pollock BE, Driscoll CL, Link MJ. Significance of cochlear dose in the radiosurgical treatment of vestibular schwannoma: controversies and unanswered questions. *Neurosurgery*. 2014 May;74(5):466-74; discussion 474.

[35] van Linge A, van Os R, Hoekstra N, Heijmen B, Stienstra L, Dallenga A, Wolbers J, Mendez Romero A. Progression of hearing

loss after LINAC-based stereotactic radiotherapy for vestibular schwannoma is associated with cochlear dose, not with pre-treatment hearing level. *Radiat Oncol.* 2018 Dec 24;13(1):253.

[36] Apicella, G., Paolini, M., Deantonio, L., Masini, L., Krengli, M. Radiotherapy for vestibular schwannoma: Review of recent literature results. *Rep Pract Oncol Radiother.* 2016 Jul-Aug; 21(4):399-406.

[37] Thomas, C., Di Maio, S., Ma, R., Vollans, E., Chu, C., Clark, B., Lee, R., McKenzie, M., Martin, M., Toyota, B. Hearing preservation following fractionated stereotactic radiotherapy for vestibular schwannomas: prognostic implications of cochlear dose. *J Neurosurg.* 2007 Nov;107(5):917-26.

[38] Kopp, C., Fauser, C., Müller, A., Astner, S. T., Jacob, V., Lumenta, C., Meyer B, Tonn JC, Molls M, Grosu AL. Stereotactic fractionated radiotherapy and LINAC radiosurgery in the treatment of vestibular schwannoma-report about both stereotactic methods from a single institution. *Int J Radiat Oncol Biol Phys.* 2011 Aug 1;80(5):1485-91.

[39] Collen, C., Ampe, B., Gevaert T., Moens, M., Linthout, N., De Ridder, M., Verellen, D., D'Haens, J., Storme, G. Single fraction versus fractionated linac-based stereotactic radiotherapy for vestibular schwannoma: a single-institution experience. *Int J Radiat Oncol Biol Phys.* 2011 Nov 15;81(4):e503-9.

[40] Anderson, B. M., Khuntia, D., Bentzen, S. M., Geye, H. M., Hayes, L. L., Kuo, J. S., Baskaya, M. K., Badie, B., Basavatia, A., Pyle, G. M., Tomé W. A., Mehta M. P. Single institution experience treating 104 vestibular schwannomas with fractionated stereotactic radiation therapy or stereotactic radiosurgery. *J Neurooncol.* 2014 Jan;116(1): 187-93.

[41] Woolf, D. K., Williams M., Goh, C. L., Henderson, D. R., Menashy, R. V., Simpson, N., Mastroianni, B., Collis, C. H. Fractionated stereotactic radiotherapy for acoustic neuromas: long-term outcomes. *Clin Oncol* (R Coll Radiol). 2013 Dec; 25(12):734-8.

[42] Litre, F., Rousseaux, P., Jovenin, N., Bazin, A., Peruzzi, P., Wdowczyk, D., Colin, P. Fractionated stereotactic radiotherapy for

acoustic neuromas: a prospective monocenter study of about 158 cases. *Radiother Oncol.* 2013 Feb;106(2):169-74.

[43] Champ C. E., Shen X., Shi W., Mayekar S. U., Chapman K., Werner-Wasik, M., Farrell, C. J., Gunn, V., Downes, M. B., Liu, H., Evans, J. J., Andrews, D. W. Reduced-dose fractionated stereotactic radiotherapy for acoustic neuromas: maintenance of tumor control with improved hearing preservation. *Neurosurgery.* 2013 Sep;73(3): 489-96.

[44] Williams, B. J., Xu, Z., Salvetti, D. J., McNeill, I. T., Larner, J., Sheehan, J. P. Gamma Knife surgery for large vestibular schwannomas: a single-center retrospective case-matched comparison assessing the effect of lesion size. *J Neurosurg.* 2013 Aug;119(2):463-71.

[45] Meijer O. W., Vandertop W. P., Baayen J. C., Slotman B. J. Single-fraction vs. fractionated linac-based stereotactic radiosurgery for vestibular schwannoma: a single-institution study. *Int J Radiat Oncol Biol Phys.* 2003 Aug 1;56(5):1390-6.

[46] Mahboubi H, Sahyouni R, Moshtaghi O, Tadokoro K, Ghavami Y, Ziai K, Lin HW, Djalilian HR. CyberKnife for Treatment of Vestibular Schwannoma: A Meta-analysis. *Otolaryngol Head Neck Surg.* 2017 Jul;157(1):7-15.

[47] Chang, S. D., Gibbs, I. C., Sakamoto, G. T., Lee, E., Oyelese, A., Adler Jr., J. R. Staged stereotactic irradiation for acoustic neuroma. *Neurosurgery.* 2005 Jun;56(6):1254-61; discussion 1261-3.

[48] Hansasuta A, Choi CY, Gibbs IC, Soltys SG, Tse VC, Lieberson RE, Hayden MG, Sakamoto GT, Harsh GR 4th, Adler JR Jr, Chang SD. Multisession stereotactic radiosurgery for vestibular schwannomas: single-institution experience with 383 cases. *Neurosurgery.* 2011 Dec;69(6):1200-9.

[49] Tsai J. T., Lin J. W., Lin C. M., Chen Y. H., Ma H. I., Jen Y. M., Chen, Y. H., Ju, D. T. Clinical evaluation of CyberKnife in the treatment of vestibular schwannomas. *Biomed Res Int.* 2013;2013: 297093.

[50] Amichetti M, Amelio D, Minniti G. Radiosurgery with photons or protons for benign and malignant tumours of the skull base: a review. *Radiat Oncol.* 2012 Dec 14;7:210.

[51] Weber, D. C., Chan, A. W., Bussiere, M. R., Harsh, G. R. 4th, Ancukiewicz, M, Barker, FG 2nd, Thornton, AT, Martuza, R. L., Nadol Jr., J. B., Chapman, P. H., Loeffler, J. S. Proton beam radiosurgery for vestibular schwannoma: tumor control and cranial nerve toxicity. *Neurosurgery.* 2003 Sep;53(3):577-86; discussion 586-8.

[52] Bush, D. A., McAllister C. J., Loredo L. N., Johnson W. D., Slater, J. M., Slater J. D. Fractionated proton beam radiotherapy for acoustic neuroma. *Neurosurgery.* 2002 Feb;50(2):270-3; discussion 273-5.

[53] Vernimmen, F. J., Mohamed, Z., Slabbert, J. P., Wilson, J. Long-term results of stereotactic proton beam radiotherapy for acoustic neuromas. *Radiother Oncol.* 2009 Feb;90(2):208-12.

In: Vestibular Schwannoma
Editors: Francesco Dispenza et al.
ISBN: 978-1-53617-191-4

Chapter 12

FACIAL NERVE RESTORATION AFTER VESTIBULAR SCHWANNOMA SURGERY

S. Taliente[1], M. Maruccia[2], R. Guarino[1], R. Elia[2], G. Giudice[2] and Nicola Quaranta[1]

[1]Division of Otolaryngology, Department of BMS, Neuroscience and Sensory Organs University of Bari, Bari, Italy
[2]Division of Plastic and Reconstructive Surgery, Department of Emergency and Organ Transplantation, University of Bari, Bari, Italy

ABSTRACT

Facial nerve (FN) palsy represents the most frequent complication of VS surgery, therefore all of the professionals involved in the treatment of VS should be aware of its implications and treatment. Several treatments have been described for the management of facial nerve paralysis. The choice of the repair technique depends on various factors, including the type and site of lesion, the time elapsed from the injurious event, the patient's expectations and the rehabilitation. Post-operative facial nerve paralysis can be treated with static and dynamic techniques.

Static techniques are based on the passive correction of muscle deficits without restoring their movement, while dynamic techniques aim to restore the active function of the affected mimic muscles, through the restoration of the muscular innervation or their replacement with free or pedunculated muscle flaps.

INTRODUCTION

Vestibular Schwannoma (VS) is one of the most difficult brain tumours to remove. They account for the 85-92% of cerebellopontine angle tumours, 93.1% of intracranial nerve Schwann cell tumour and 7.79-19.64%, of intracranial tumours [1].

Over the past 25 years VS surgery has undergone immense changes and the progressive improvement of surgical instruments and techniques have drastically reduced the mortality rate [2].

The focus of the surgery has passed from the preservation of "life" to the preservation of "quality of life" with more attention to the preservation of the cranial nerves function.

Facial nerve (FN) palsy represents the most frequent complication of VS surgery, therefore all of the professionals involved in the treatment of VS should be aware of its implications and treatment [3].

The effect of FN palsy are both clinical and psychological. From a clinical point of view facial palsy induces oral incompetence, collapse of the nasal valve, dysfunctional lacrimation up to possible serious ophthalmic complications like corneal ulceration [4] while the loss of facial expression and the alteration of the muscular tone and movements reduce significantly the quality of life of these patients [5].

The treatment of VS has changed in the last 20 years; small tumours are managed conservatively, while surgery is reserved for medium-large sized VS and radiologically growing tumours [6].

In VS surgery the facial nerve is at high risk of lesion due to its intimate relationship with the tumour. The introduction of the operating microscope by William House [7] and the use of facial nerve neurophysiological monitoring [8] has considerably decreased the incidence of postoperative facial palsy [6, 9].

However, facial nerve outcome after VS surgery is influenced by several factors and the size of the tumours represents the most important one [1, 10]. Additional factors that can influence the prognosis of FN function have been reported, such as the patient's age and comorbidities, the extent of tumour removal (complete vs partial removal), the gross anatomy of the tumour (cystic vs non cystic form) [10].

CLASSIFICATION AND TREATMENT

Several classifications have been proposed to categorize facial nerve function such as the FaCE Scale [11], the Facial Disability Index [FDI] [12], Sunnybrook's staging system [13]; still, the most utilized classification is the House-Brackmann grading system [14].

In 2003 Kanzaki et al. [15] proposed a modification of the HB scale for reporting facial nerve outcome after VS surgery (Table 1).

Several treatments have been described for the management of facial nerve paralysis. The choice of the repair technique depends on various factors, including the type and site of lesion, the time elapsed from the injurious event, the patient's expectations and the rehabilitation possibilities [16].

Facial Nerve paralysis after VS surgery can immediate or delayed.

- Immediate paralysis is related to intraoperative trauma of the nerve. In case the nerve is intact and responds to intraoperative electrical stimulation, a post-operative palsy is treated with post-operative steroids (e.g., dexamethasone i. v. at 4 mg every 6 hours during 48 hours).

Table 1. Kanzaki et al. Tokyo Classification

Grade I		**Normal facial function in all areas**
Grade II	Gross:-	Slight weakness noticeable on close inspection
	Synkinesis*	Very slight-noticeable on close inspection when the mouth is protruded forcibly
	At rest:-	Normal symmetry and tone
	Motions:	a) Forehead: Moderate to good function
		b) Eye: complete closure with minimal effort
		c) Mouth: Slight asymmetry
Grade III A	Gross:-	Obvious but not disfiguring difference between th two sides.
	Synkinesis*	*Slight* noticeable but not complete when the mouth protruded forcibly. Some contracture and/or hemifacial spasm may be present.
	At rest:-	Normal symmetry and tone
	Motions:	a) Forehead: slight to moderate movements
		b) Eye: complete closure with effort *eye comfortable and in good condition with or without lubricants*
		c) Mouth: Weak with maximum effort
Grade III B	Gross:-	Obvious but not disfiguring difference between the two sides.
	Synkinesis*	*Moderate* eye close completely when the mouth is protruded forcibly some contracture and/or hemifacial spasm may be present
	At rest:-	Normal symmetry and tone
	Motions:	a) Forehead: slight to moderate movements
		b) Eye: complete closure with effort *eye dry and uncomfortable with evidence of exposure keratitis requiring lucricants and possibly tarsorrhaphy*
		c) Mouth: Weak with maximum effort
Grade IV	Gross:-	Obvious weakness and disfiguring asymmetry
	Synkinesis*	*Severe*_- Apparent mass motion whilst speaking
	At rest:-	Normal symmetry and tone
	Motions:	a) Forehead: None
		b) Eye: incomplete closure
		c) Mouth: Asymmetry with maximum effort
Grade V	Gross:-	Barely perceptible or no motion
	At rest:-	Asymmetry
	Motions:	a) Forehead: none
		b) Eye: none or incomplete closure
		c) Mouth: Slight or no movement
Grade VI		No movement. No tone.

* Synkinesis can be assessed by observed the degree of the eye closure when the mouth moves or by forcible protrusion of the lips. Synkinesis may include contracture and/or hemifacial spasm.

In cases of intraoperative interruption of the nerve, immediate reconstruction gives the best long term results [17] (see below).

- Occasionally a *delayed paralysis* can present several days after the surgery. High-dose of steroids are indicated and recovery is possible in most cases [18].

Facial Nerve Repair Techniques

- Intraoperative repair

In case of intraoperative interruption of the nerve immediate reconstruction is indicated, being direct end-to-end anastomosis the preferred technique [18].

- Direct end-to-end anastomosis (or primary neurorrhaphy)

Direct end-to-end anastomosis (or primary neurorrhaphy) is considered the best option in case of acute post-traumatic facial nerve palsy in terms of recovery outcomes [19, 20].

After the removal of the VS, nerve stumps are identified and brought together. It is essential to avoid any tension between the two nerve stumps (proximal and distal), and to have a sufficient and useful contact between the endoneural surfaces. No difference has been shown between epineural and fascicular repair in terms of functional result in case of monofascicular nerve stumps. In polyfascicular nerve stumps, an interfascicular repair secures an optimal alignment of the nerve ends. Nerve repair is carried out using non-resorbable 8-10/0 suture.

To avoid tension between the two stumps in translabyrinthine surgery it is possible to free the second and third portion of the nerve from its bony channel and reroute it in the cerebellopontine angle where the two stumps are anastomosed. Since direct suturing, especially in the cerebello-pontine angle, is most of the time difficult, fibrin glue and temporalis fascia can be used instead of sutures [21].

- Interposition nerve grafts

When the nerve anastomosis cannot be performed without tension or there is a nerve gap, an interposition (or cable) nerve graft is used.

The sural nerve, the great auricular nerve or the medial antebrachial cutaneous nerve are the most common donor sites of nerve grafts because they are long, unbranched and they are not associated with critical sensory deficit. Both sides of the nerve graft is co-opted in an end-to-end fashion to the ends of the two stumps. Also in this case the fibrin glue and fascia are used instead of sutures.

Immediate repair of the facial nerve leads to HB grade 3 in most of the cases [22].

Post-Operative Facial Nerve Rehabilitation

Post-operative facial nerve paralysis can be treated with static and dynamic techniques.

Static techniques are based on the passive correction of muscle deficits without restoring their movement, while dynamic techniques aim to restore the active function of the affected mimic muscles, through the restoration of the muscular innervation or their replacement with free or pedunculated muscle flaps.

Static Reanimation

Static reanimation is used to achieve symmetry or a slightly overcorrection at rest on the normal side without providing animation. Static procedures are a good option for repairing specific cosmetic or functional deficits of the peri-orbital, perioral and to address nasal obstruction due to nasal valve collapse [22].

Although dynamic reanimation should be the gold standard, in a subset of patients, static techniques may be more appropriate. For patients with significant comorbidities, a shortened life span, advanced age, patients who are not good candidates for prolonged general anaesthesia, or in whom free muscle transfer may not be appropriate, static correction can still provide improved symmetry and function [23].

Rehabilitating the eye is one of the most important immediate needs in facial paralysis. Paralytic lower eyelid ectropion/retraction and lack of upper eyelid closure contribute to lagophthalmos and lacrimal dysfunction. A gold or platinum weight can be placed in a submuscolar pocket along the superior margin of the tarsal plate (Figure 1). Other techniques to improve the paralyzed eye include tarsorrhaphy, lateral canthopexy; a modification of a tarsoconjunctival flap has also been described to repair ectropion and lagofhtalmos [24, 25].

Functional deficits related to midface flaccidity include external nasal valve collapse and nasal obstruction, and lip ptosis with associated drooling and speech difficulty. The entire midface cheek complex also becomes ptotic and displaced inferiorly exacerbating lower eyelid and lip ptosis.

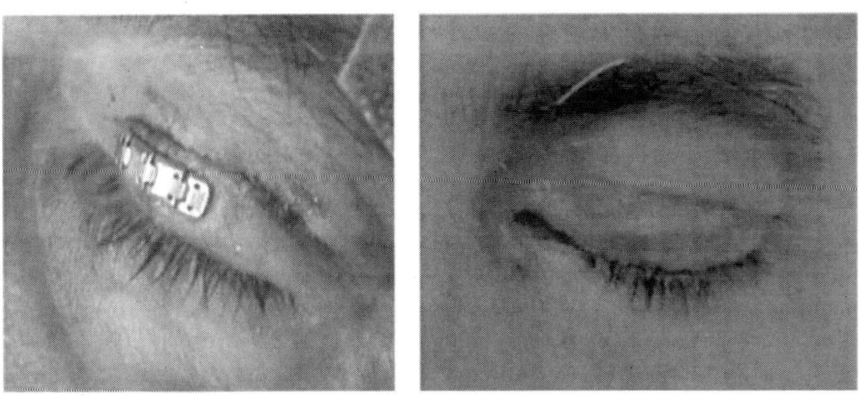

Figure 1. Gold weight. Note the gold weight on the upper eyelid, placed at a submuscolar pocket along the superior margin of the tarsal plate.

Static suspension with slings can be used. Slings can be made of fascia (tensor fascia latae), tendon (palmaris longus) or prosthetic material such as Gore-Tex®. The graft is attached to the temporal fascia or to the zygoma. Midface subperiostal lifts may also be beneficial.

Dynamic Reanimation

The aims of a dynamic procedure are to restore voluntary movement, especially the smile, resting tone and facial symmetry.

Reconstructive modalities for facial paralysis can be classified by two basic criteria: the first is whether the reconstruction is based on the facial nerve or on a different cranial nerve and the second is whether the working muscle unit is the original facial musculature or a transferred muscle flap.

Reanimation based on the facial nerve can be on the ipsilateral or contralateral nerve depending on the presence of a functional and usable branch or stump. The duration of paralysis is the determinant for the need for muscle transfer or transplant: if it is less than 12 months, the facial musculature is assumed to be able to be reinnervated. Muscles become irreversibly atrophic by 24 months, in which case muscle replacement is indicated. Even if surgical techniques for dynamic nervous resuscitation have been improved in the recent years, it is still very difficult to obtain an House Brackmann grade better than grade 3 [26].

Reinnervation

The aim of reinnervation procedures is to re-establish the input to facial nerve stumps using donors other than the native facial nerve. This procedure is useful when the proximal stump of the nerve is no longer available for example in very large tumours with distorted anatomy.

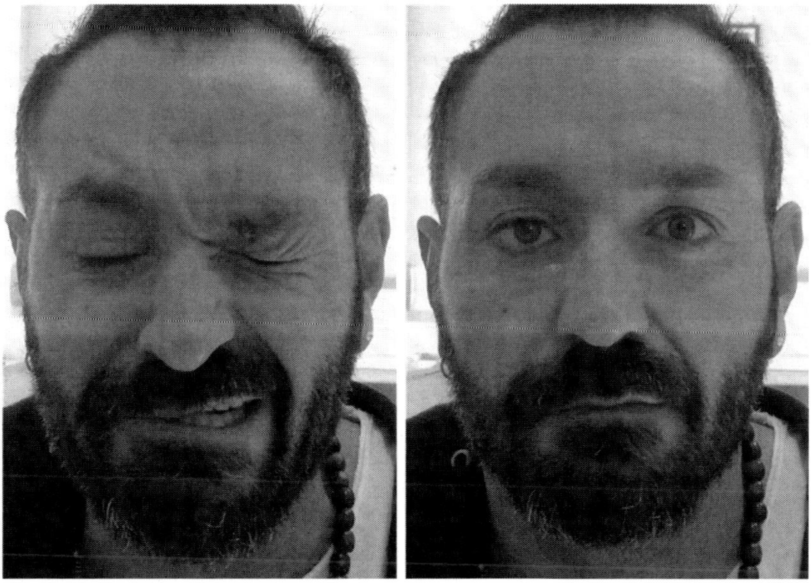

Figure 2. Hypoglossal-to-facial nerve transfer (post-operative result). A HB grade III is achieved (note the complete closure of the right eye) at 12 months of follow up.

Hypoglossal (XII) - to - Facial (VII) Nerve Transfer

The VII nerve is identified at the stylomastoid foramen and transected, while the XII nerve is divided distally, reflected upward and sutured with the VII nerve. Alternatively the XII nerve is partially divided in order to avoid tongue atrophy and a great auricular nerve "jump graft" can be coopted between the XII and the VII nerve. In this case an end-to-side anastomosis is performed, although a tongue dysfunction may occur in the 25% of the patients and the transfer may lead to an unnatural appearing activation of the intact facial musculature [27, 28].

After 12-months an HB grade 3 with synkinesis can be achieved (Figure 2).

Masseter to Facial Nerve Transfer

Masseterine nerve (or the masseteric branch of the trigeminal nerve) has become most recently a good donor site to innervate facial musculature because of its anatomic location, relative easy dissection and the facial nerve results [4, 29, 30].

VII-VII Cross Facial Nerve Grafting (CFNG)

The CFNG technique uses branches of contralateral functioning facial nerve to innervate paralyzed muscles. A nerve graft (e.g., sural nerve graft) connects healthy peripheral nerve branches to corresponding branches of specific muscle groups on paralyzed sides. CFNG can be performed as one stage or two-stages procedure. In the first stage the selectively neurectomized branches of the unaffected facial nerve provide motor fibers through CFNGs; after 9-12 months and after electrophysiological confirmation, secondary microcoaptation takes place with corresponding branches of the affected facial nerve. If denervation is longer than 6 months, a partial hypoglossal-to-facial nerve graft can be combined to CFNG two-stages procedure to prevent atrophy and loss of motor endplates ('babysitter' of the facial muscles, as described by Terzis [31]).

Local Muscle Transposition

Muscle transposition is performed when there is irreversible muscolar atrophy and fibrosis, due to the long denervation period.

Temporalis Muscle Transfer

It is still considered the best choice for facial rehabilitation due to the greater excursion of movement and adaptability to orbit. The muscle with its fascial extensions can be transferred and sutured to eyelids, ala of nose, oral commissure, and upper and lower lips. Labbè et al. [32] described a lengthening myoplasty: the tendon is rerouted to the corner of the mouth and additional length is achieved by repositioning the muscle's origin on the skull.

Masseter Muscle Transfer

It is a valuable option for the rehabilitation of the buccal complex. It is possible to recover an acceptable smile, a raising of the upper lip and the buccal angle. The muscle is, indeed, released from the mandible and transposed to the orbicularis oris resulting in a lateral vector.

Digastric Muscle Transfer

The anterior digastric tendon is mobilized and inserted into orbicularis oris at inferior vermilion border. The technique can be applied in case of isolated mandibular branch palsy to restore lower lip depression function.

Microneurovascular Muscle Transposition

The microneurovascular muscle transfer is indicated in case of long-standing facial paralysis, when facial muscles cannot gain useful function after reinnervation. The main advantage of a free functional muscle transfer vs local muscle transfer is the possibility to control precisely the origin, insertion, tension and location of the muscle. The procedure can be performed in one stage if the motor nerve is directly sutured to a branch of the contralateral facial nerve. The functional improvement is visible within few months, avoiding nerve grafts and a second operation. Nevertheless, there is a lack of suitable muscle (long neurovascular bundle), except for children. The two stage procedure involves a CFNG before harvesting a free muscle flap.

The following muscles may be used as free functioning transfers:

- Gracilis muscle: it is considered the gold standard for rehabilitating the oral commissure [16, 33-35] (Figure 3)
- Pectoralis minor
- Latissimus dorsi muscle, that allows recovery of facial symmetry, muscle tone and expression similar to the traditional temporalis muscle transfer [36]
- Serratus anterior
- Rectus abdominis
- Rectus femoris
- Sartorius
- Abductor hallucis.

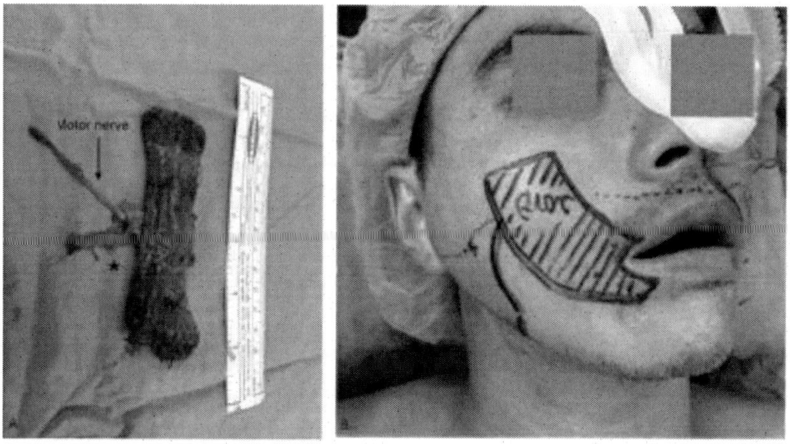

Figure 3. Free gracilis muscle transfer for smile restoration (intraoperative views). A. Harvest of free gracilis muscle flap. The photograph shows the dominant vascular pedicle (asterisk) and the gracilis motor nerve. Note the marker sutures placed at 1cm intervals, to insert the muscle at the in situ tension. B. Scheme of the free gracilis muscle flap inset. The muscle is transferred to the cheek pocket. The vascular pedicle is anastomosed to the facial vessels and the motor nerve coaptation is made to the masseteric nerve.

CONCLUSION

The aim of vestibular schwannoma surgery is total tumour removal with the preservation of the facial nerve integrity and minimal postoperative morbidity.

If a facial reanimation is necessary, immediate nerve repair yields the best outcomes.

If the denervation time is less than 12-18 months, facial muscle can be reinnervated through reinnervation procedures.

If the denervation is over 24 months, CFNGs are used for neurotization of free or pedicled vascularized muscle transfer for facial muscle substitution (Figure 4).

Revision and ancillary procedures along with early and long term follow up are essential to determine the functional and aesthetic outcome.

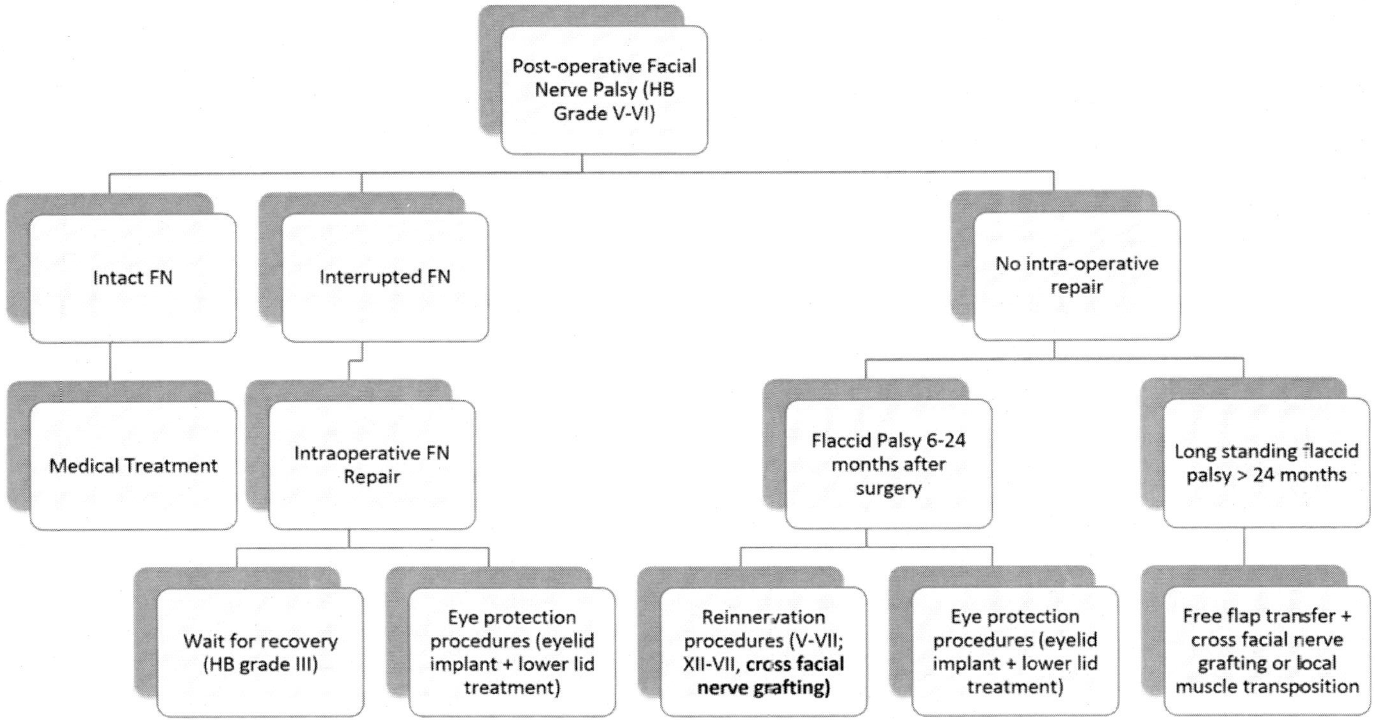

Figure 4. Facial reanimation treatment algorithm.

REFERENCES

[1] Samii M, Matthies C. Management of 1000 vestibular schwannomas (acoustic neuromas): surgical management and results with an emphasis on complications and how to avoid them. *Neurosurgery*. 1997;40(1):11-21.

[2] Falcioni M, Fois P, Taibah A, Sanna M. Facial nerve function after vestibular schwannoma surgery. *J. Neurosurg*. 2011;115(4):820-826.

[3] Dandinarasaiah M, Prasad SC, Piccirillo E, et al. Facial Nerve Outcomes Following Total Excision of Vestibular Schwannoma by the Enlarged Translabyrinthine Approach. *Otol. Neurotol. Off Publ. Am. Otol. Soc. Am. Neurotol. Soc. Eur. Acad. Otol. Neurotol*. 2019;40(2):226-235.

[4] Hadlock TA, Cheney ML, McKenna MJ, Facial reanimation surgery. In: Nadol Jr JP, Mckenna MJ editors. *Surgery of the ear and temporal bone*. Philadelphia (PA). Lippincott Williams and Wilkins; 2005. pp 461-472.

[5] Dey JK, Ishii LE, Byrne PJ, Boahene KDO, Ishii M. Seeing is believing: objectively evaluating the impact of facial reanimation surgery on social perception. *The Laryngoscope*. 2014;124(11):2489-2497.

[6] Sampath P, Holliday MJ, Brem H, Niparko JK, Long DM. Facial nerve injury in acoustic neuroma (vestibular schwannoma) surgery: etiology and prevention. *J. Neurosurg*. 1997;87(1):60-66.

[7] House WF. Acoustic neuroma. Case summaries. *Arch. Otolaryngol. Chic. Ill.* 1960. 1968;88(6):586-591.

[8] Delgado TE, Bucheit WA, Rosenholtz HR, Chrissian S. Intraoperative monitoring of facila muscle evoked responses obtained by intracranial stimulation of the facila nerve: a more accurate technique for facila nerve dissection. *Neurosurgery*. 1979;4(5):418-421.

[9] Nicoli F, D'Ambrosia C, Lazzeri D, et al. Microsurgical dissection of facial nerve in parotidectomy: a discussion of techniques and long-term results. *Gland Surg*. 2017;6(4):308-314.

[10] Grey PL, Moffat DA, Palmer CR, Hardy DG, Baguley DM. Factors which influence the facial nerve outcome in vestibular schwannoma surgery. *Clin. Otolaryngol. Allied Sci*. 1996;21(5):409-413.

[11] Kahn JB, Gliklich RE, Boyev KP, Stewart MG, Metson RB, McKenna MJ. Validation of a patient-graded instrument for facial nerve paralysis: the FaCE scale. *The Laryngoscope*. 2001;111(3):387-398.

[12] Van Swearingen JM, Brach JS. The Facial Disability Index: reliability and validity of a disability assessment instrument for disorders of the facial neuromuscular system. *Phys. Ther*. 1996;76(12):1288-1298.

[13] Neely JG, Cherian NG, Dickerson CB, Nedzelski JM. Sunnybrook facial grading system: reliability and criteria for grading. *The Laryngoscope*. 2010;120(5):1038-1045.

[14] House JW, Brackmann DE. Facial nerve grading system. *Otolaryngol. - Head Neck Surg. Off J. Am. Acad. Otolaryngol. - Head Neck Surg*. 1985;93(2):146-147.

[15] Kanzaki J, Tos M, Sanna M, Moffat DA, Monsell EM, Berliner KI. New and modified reporting systems from the consensus meeting on systems for reporting results in vestibular schwannoma. *Otol. Neurotol. Off Publ. Am. Otol. Soc. Am. Neurotol. Soc. Eur. Acad. Otol. Neurotol*. 2003;24(4):642-648.

[16] Boahene K. Facial reanimation after acoustic neuroma resection: options and timing of intervention. *Facial Plast. Surg. FPS*. 2015;31(2):103-109.

[17] Mehta RP. Surgical treatment of facial paralysis. *Clin. Exp. Otorhinolaryngol*. 2009;2(1):1-5.

[18] Slattery III WH, Brandt M. Acoustic Neuromas and Facial Paralysis. In: *The facial nerve*. pp 155-163 (chapter 20) Ed. Thieme 2014.

[19] Bailey BJ, Johnson JT, Newlands SD. *Head & Neck Surgery - Otolaryngology*. Philadelphia, PA: Lippincott Williams & Wilkins; 2006.

[20] Divi V, Deschler DG. Re-animation and rehabilitation of the paralyzed face in head and neck cancer patients. *Clin. Anat. N Y N.* 2012;25(1):99-107.

[21] Sanna M, Khrais T, Mancini F et al. Facial Nerve Reanimation. In: *The facial nerve in temporal bone and lateral skull base microsurgery*. 2006, cap 5; pp 43-60

[22] Prasad SC, Balasubramanian K, Piccirillo E, et al. Surgical technique and results of cable graft interpositioning of the facial nerve in lateral skull base surgeries: experience with 213 consecutive cases. *J. Neurosurg*. 2018;128(2):631-638.

[23] Lafer MP, O TM. Management of Long-Standing Flaccid Facial Palsy: Static Approaches to the Brow, Midface, and Lower Lip. *Otolaryngol. Clin. North Am.* 2018;51(6):1141-1150.

[24] Sufyan AS, Lee HBH, Shah H, Nunery WR, Kokoska MS, Shipchandler TZ. Single-stage repair of paralytic ectropion using a novel modification of the tarsoconjunctival flap. *JAMA Facial Plast. Surg*. 2014;16(2):151-152.

[25] Homer N, Fay A. Management of Long-Standing Flaccid Facial Palsy: Periocular Considerations. *Otolaryngol. Clin. North Am.* 2018;51(6):1107-1118.

[26] Rabie AN, Ibrahim AMS, Kim PS, et al. Dynamic rehabilitation of facial nerve injury: a review of the literature. *J. Reconstr. Microsurg*. 2013;29(5):283-296.

[27] Viterbo F, Amr AH, Stipp EJ, Reis FJ. End-to-side neurorrhaphy: past, present, and future. *Plast. Reconstr. Surg*. 2009;124(6 Suppl):e351-358.

[28] Darrouzet V, Dutkiewicz J, Chambrin A, Stoll D, Bébéar JP. [Hypoglosso-facial anastomosis: results and technical development towards end-to-side anastomosis with rerouting of the intra-temporal facial nerve (modified May technique)]. *Rev. Laryngol. - Otol. - Rhinol*. 1997;118(3):203-210.

[29] Henstrom DK. Masseteric nerve use in facial reanimation. *Curr. Opin. Otolaryngol. Head Neck Surg*. 2014;22(4):284-290.

[30] Klebuc MJA. Facial reanimation using the masseter-to-facial nerve transfer. *Plast. Reconstr. Surg*. 2011;127(5):1909-1915.

[31] Terzis JK, Tzafetta K. The "babysitter" procedure: minihypoglossal to facial nerve transfer and cross-facial nerve grafting. *Plast. Reconstr. Surg*. 2009;123(3):865-876.

[32] Labbé D, Huault M. Lengthening temporalis myoplasty and lip reanimation. *Plast. Reconstr. Surg*. 2000;105(4):1289-1297.

[33] Harris BN, Tollefson TT. Facial reanimation: evolving from static procedures to free tissue transfer in head and neck surgery. *Curr. Opin. Otolaryngol. Head Neck Surg*. 2015;23(5):399-406.

[34] Ciudad P, Agko M, Manrique OJ, et al. The retrograde transverse cervical artery as a recipient vessel for free tissue transfer in complex head and neck reconstruction with a vessel-depleted neck. *Microsurgery*. 2017;37(8):902-909.

[35] Nicoli F, Chilgar RM, Sapountzis S, et al. Reconstruction after orbital exenteration using gracilis muscle free flap. *Microsurgery*. 2015;35(3):169-176.

[36] Tate JR, Tollefson TT. Advances in facial reanimation. *Curr. Opin. Otolaryngol. Head Neck Surg*. 2006;14(4):242-248.

In: Vestibular Schwannoma
Editors: Francesco Dispenza et al.
ISBN: 978-1-53617-191-4

Chapter 13

VESTIBULAR AND PROPRIOCEPTIVE REHABILITATION STRATEGY IN ACOUSTIC NEURINOMA

Valerio Giustino[1], MSc, Federico Sireci[2], MD, Giulia Letizia Mauro[3], MD, Giuseppe Messina[4,5], MD, Serena Rizzo[3], MD and Francesco Martines[2], MD, PhD

[1]PhD Program in Health Promotion and Cognitive Sciences, University of Palermo, Palermo, Italy
[2]Bi.N.D. Department, University of Palermo, Audiology Section, Palermo, Italy
[3]University of Palermo, Di.Chir.On.S. Department, Section of Physical Medicine and Rehabilitation, Palermo, Italy
[4]Department of Psychology, Educational Science and Human Movement, University of Palermo, Palermo, Italy
[5]PosturaLab Italia Research Institute, Palermo, Italy

ABSTRACT

Rehabilitation therapy can be used to treat balance disorders via exercises organized into anatomo-pathological protocols. In general, there is an indication for rehabilitation whenever compensation of a patient's vestibular system fails to adequately resolve spontaneously. Although the therapeutical indications have expanded over time, it is especially useful to treat balance disorders in neurological patients and those with acute damage to the vestibular system. Specifically, it favors and accelerates spontaneous central compensation in a variety of neurological disorders such as Multiple Sclerosis, Parkinson's disease, cerebellar pathologies or in brain tumors like Vestibular Schwannoma (or Acoustic Neurinoma). The latter is a benign intracranial tumor that affects the acoustic nerve (or cranial nerve VIII), which is concerned with hearing, balance and head position. It represents about 6% of all intracranial tumors, with an incidence of approximately 1 per 100,000 person-years. Affected patients present with a range of symptoms including discomfort, reduced motor capacity and afflictions that lead to functional limitations in the activities of daily life and personal care, especially in performing tasks requiring some degree of postural balance. The aim is to treat them through a series of exercises to be repeated both with the aid of a specialized supervisor and unassisted at home; the treatment is based on proprioceptive and vestibular exercises that progressively improve their quality of life.

Keywords: Vestibular Schwannoma, risk of falls, postural control, posture and balance

1. INTRODUCTION

Vestibular Schwannoma (VS), commonly known as Acoustic Neuroma, is a benign and usually slow-growing tumor. It develops on the vestibulocochlear nerve (cranial nerve VIII), specifically from the Schwann cells responsible for myelin sheath production, which maintains peripheral nerves insulated. It represents about 6% of all intracranial tumors, with an incidence of approximately 1 per 100,000 person-years [1, 2]. VS patients are typically diagnosed between 50 and 60 years of age. Prevalence data show no significant differences among sexes or preference with respect to laterality [3, 4]. Although many potential causes of VS have been extensively evaluated, most cases elude a definitive etiology. Nevertheless, several studies have shown various predisposing factors for the development of VS, such as ionizing radiation, radio frequency electromagnetic fields (e.g., from mobile phone use), noise exposure and allergies. Studies regarding pediatric atomic-bomb survivors in Japan have shown a correlation between moderate to high doses of ionizing radiation and an increased incidence of VS [5, 6, 7]. Signs and symptoms of VS are often elusive and may require many years to appear. The latter often impair hearing and balance reflecting its origin from cranial nerve VIII. Subjects typically have: disturbances of static and dynamic postural control with far less frequent relapsing objective rotatory vertigo [8]; hearing loss, usually of slow onset, but at times sudden [9], general occurs, or is more prominent, on the affected side; tinnitus (an annoyingly persistent or recurring perception of a ringing or buzzing in the ear) on the affected side; paresthesias of facial muscles, loss of facial mimicry and, in more severe cases, facial nerve palsy.

Occasionally they also report feeling uneasy in new or unfamiliar settings, increasing their risk of falls. These afflictions may significantly impair a patient's autonomy and social well-being, as well as hinder their daily activities. Our aim is to provide patients with an effective multidisciplinary approach, starting with a timely and accurate diagnosis.

2. Etiology

A causal role of VS appears to arise from a defective gene on chromosome 22. Physiologically, this gene produces a tumor-suppressor protein that helps control the growth of Schwann cells that line the axons. The reasons for the gene malfunction have yet to be elucidated and the cause in most cases of VS remains unknown. Indeed, although many potential causes of VS have been reported, no definitive etiology can be identified in many cases despite thorough evaluations. However, several studies have shown some VS risk factors, such as ionizing radiation, radio frequency electromagnetic fields (e.g., from mobile phone use), excessive noise exposure and allergies. Studies in pediatric Japanese age atomic-bomb survivors have shown a correlation between moderate to high doses of ionizing radiation and an increased incidence of VS [5, 6, 7]. This faulty gene is also present in Neurofibromatosis type 2 (NF2). It is a rare autosomal dominant disorder (incidence 1:33,000-40,000) characterized by central nervous system tumors and mutation in the NF2 gene on chromosome 22q12. VSs, typically bilateral, are the hallmark lesion, affecting approximately 95% of individuals.

3. DIAGNOSIS

Diagnosing VS is often challenging, especially in its early stages because signs and symptoms may be subtle and develop gradually over time. Of note, hearing loss and dizziness are also non-specific symptoms associated with a variety of other middle and inner ear conditions.

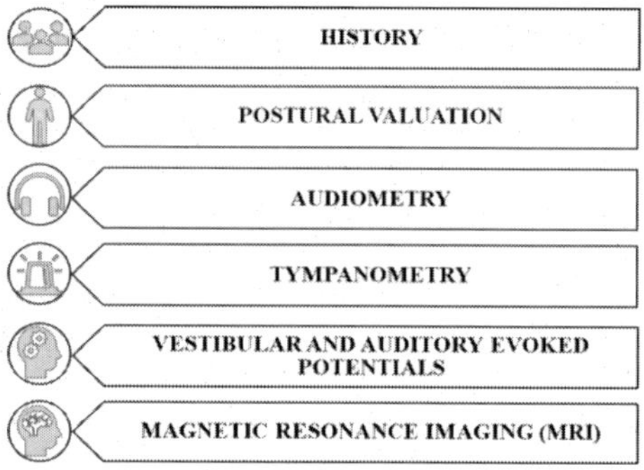

Figure 1. Diagnostic flowchart in vestibular schwannoma

The mainstays of the diagnostic approach comprise (Figure 1): history, postural evaluation, audiometry, tympanometry (including stapedial reflex testing), vestibular and auditory evoked potentials, as well as Magnetic Resonance Imaging (MRI).

The typical history, per se, seldom makes for a straightforward diagnosis. Clinicians should focus on the accompanying circumstances, pattern of symptom onset and temporal progression.

Postural evaluation [10, 11, 12, 13] is performed by way of several tests: Romberg Test, Fukuda Test, Walking Test, always giving due consideration to static standing posture on a force platform.

Hearing Test [14, 15]. In this examination, the audiologist (hearing specialist) presents a scale of sounds of different pure tones. Each tone is repeated at increasingly lower hearing-level scales, to estimate hearing thresholds.

For a more in-depth assessment, Vestibular Evoked Myogenic Potential (VEMP) testing is also performed on the cervical musculature (cVEMP) in combination with Auditory Brainstem Response (ABR) testing.

Imaging has a key role in screening, initial and follow-up assessment of VS. Magnetic resonance imaging (MRI) is the most sensitive imaging technique to confirm the diagnosis of VS, in fact it can detect tumors as small as 1 - 2 millimeters in diameter.

If MRI is unavailable, or inappropriate for a given patient, computerized tomography (CT) may be used. The latter may however miss smaller tumors, therefore the advisability of CT should be carefully considered.

4. Signs and Symptoms

Signs and symptoms of VS are frequently subtle and of slow onset, presenting over the course of several years. They usually entail impairment of hearing and balance, as expected, given the function of the cranial nerves involved. Severe symptoms of VS may include (Figure 2):

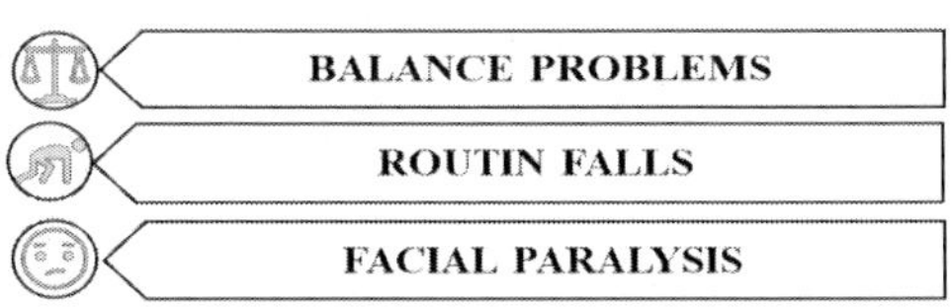

Figure 2. Signs and symptoms correlated to vestibular schwannoma

Another typical symptom is tinnitus, i.e., an annoyingly persistent, subjective perception of a ringing or buzzing sensation in the ear. Although pharmacological and non-pharmacological therapies have been proposed to treat this symptom, it commonly persists and/or recurs [16, 17].

5. Treatment

There are many treatment options for VN, the choice of which depends on several factors, mainly:

- size and position of the tumor;
- rate of growth;
- overall health conditions;

There are three fundamental treatment strategies: monitoring, surgery or radiation therapy.

6. Vestibular and Proprioceptive Rehabilitation Strategy

Falling is not simply a potentially traumatic, one-off event [18]; it may indicate an underlying impairment in the ability to maintain one's balance, typical of patients with VS. Precisely for this reason it is imperative to provide proprioceptive and vestibular rehabilitation. The purpose is to ultimately achieve optimal control of posture and balance.

Proprioceptive Rehabilitation is based on stimulation of the neuromotor system. Proprioceptive training consists of a series of exercises designed to train reflexes.

The proprioceptive training must be tailored to the situations that cause the subject to lose his or her balance, in order to quickly and effectively activate the appropriate muscles. Improvements of equilibrium occur by being able to support one's own weight unassisted while being able to quickly correct for imbalances. All proprioceptive exercises should be conducted with the patient barefoot, so as to not impede proprioceptive input from the feet.

The goal of Vestibular Rehabilitation is to overcome fear of performing movements that make the patient uneasy.

Table 1. Vestibular rehabilitation according to Cawthorne and Cooksey

The aims of the Cawthorne-Cooksey exercises include:
Relaxing the neck and shoulder muscles
Training the eyes independently of the head
Practicing the head movements that cause dizziness (to help the development of vestibular compensation)
Improving general co-ordination
Encouraging natural unprompted movement

Table 2. Goals of vestibular rehabilitation protocol

The aims of the classic protocol for vestibular rehabilitation are:
Introducing sensory substitution by increasing visual and proprioceptive inputs by improving the vestibular reflex
Enhancing vestibular plasticity
Stimulating static and dynamic balance
Promoting habituation to vertigo, instability and motor diseases
Encouraging patients to resume activities of daily living (ADLs) as soon as possible

Initially, it is recommended that patients perform the exercises under supervision and eventually repeat the exercises unassisted even at home. The first to study vestibular rehabilitation were Cawthorne and Cooksey (Table 1) [20, 21].

Based on Cawthorne and Cooksey's studies, many authors have made further contributions in drafting rehabilitation protocols (Table 2).

7. Balance Training

Various authors have suggested many other exercises. Balance training is based on the cortical capacity to analyze, memorize and reconstruct postural pose. To perform these exercises a mirror, a balancing board and a mat are indispensable (Table 3).

Table 3. Exercises for improving vertigo - Habituation Therapy

Exercises for improving vertigo (Habituation Therapy)	
Upright position, one arm above the head and the eyes look at the raised arm. Repeat on the other side. Upright position, flex the trunk until the opposite foot is touched, repeat the same movement with the opposite foot Brandt-Daroff exercise: start in an upright, seated position, move into a right or left lateral decubitus (lying) position with upturned nose at about a 45-degree angle, remain in this position for about 30 seconds (or until the vertigo subsides, whichever is longer). Then return to the sitting position. Repeat on the other side [19].	Perform 5 repetitions on each side. Perform 5 repetitions in the morning, afternoon and evening for a total time of 10 minutes, for 14 days after an episode of vertigo

The method consists in getting used to recognizing and reconstructing body position and relative position of each segment, relying both on visual control and exclusively on proprioceptive, vestibular input. Balance coordination training comprehends six phases. The patient must be able to perform all exercises correctly.

Phase 1. In front of the mirror, the patient:

- Stands with feet apart and arms outstretched
- Repeats the exercises with arms close to the body with an increasingly narrow base of support

Phase 2. In front of the mirror, the patient:

- Stands on one foot, first with eyes open, then with eyes closed
- Walks in place, first with eyes open, then with eyes closed

Phase 3. The patient:

- Walks in a straight line, first with eyes open then with eyes closed
- Walks placing one foot in front of the other (heel-to-toe), first with eyes open then with eyes closed
- Walks raising his knees, first with eyes open then with eyes closed

Phase 4. On the mat, the patient:

- Repeats all the exercises performed so far
- Gets on all fours, to perform balancing exercises

Phase 5. These exercises are initially performed with the balancing board forming a right angle to the mirror, and later with the balancing board parallel to the mirror. On the balancing board in front of the mirror, the patient:

- Progressively narrows the distance between feet

Phase 6. The patient:

- Fixes gaze on a target at eye-level and maintains visual fixation as he turns his head right and left with wide, but not excessively fast, movements
- Performs the same exercises while walking in a straight line
- Performs the same exercises while moving his head along the sagittal plane
- Performs the same exercises while moving his head as if the nose were drawing a circle around the target
- Walks in a straight-line while keeping gaze on a fixed, lateral target located at two-thirds of the distance, first on the right and then on the left

This method has many advantages: it activates central mechanisms that are rarely used in rehabilitation; patients can perform these exercises at home; and the results are evident to the subject. Moreover, this method helps patients accept their self-image and coordinate movements.

Conclusion

The aim of this chapter is to offer support in creating an individualized rehabilitative project-program for patients with Vestibular Neuroma, thus allowing them to achieve a high degree of autonomy in their lifestyle. The best strategy consists in a multidisciplinary approach, starting with the diagnosis, which addresses every facet of treatment of the various tumor-related disabilities. The secret to success is team work involving different professional figures such as physiatrists, physiotherapists, kinesiologists, neurologists and otolaryngologists. Within this multidisciplinary team, the physiatrist plays a pivotal role. The treatment is based on proprioceptive and vestibular exercises, as well as on the reduction of auditory [22, 23, 24] visual and neurological problems. Arguably, the results are always closely related to the appropriate motivational support provided by the team. Furthermore, it is essential for the patient to interact with his surroundings in order to overcome anxiety and fear, thus improving his quality of life and prognosis.

References

[1] Fisher, J. L., Pettersson, D., Palmisano, S., Schwartzbaum, J. A., Edwards, C. G., Mathiesen, T., Prochazka, M., Bergenheim, T., Florentzson, R., Harder, H., Nyberg, G., Siesjö, P., Feychting, M. (2014) Loud noise exposure and acoustic neuroma. *Am. J. Epidemiol.*, 180(1):58 - 67.

[2] Koo, M., Lai, J. T., Yang, E. Y., Liu, T. C., Hwang, J. H. (2018) Incidence of Vestibular Schwannoma in Taiwan from 2001 to 2012: A Population-Based National Health Insurance Study. *Ann. Otol. Rhinol. Laryngol.*, 127(10):694 - 697.

[3] Howitz, M. F., Johansen, C., Tos, M., Charabi, S., Olsen, J., H. (2000) Incidence of vestibular schwannoma in Denmark, 1977 - 1995. *Am. J. Otol.*, 21:690.

[4] Propp, J. M., McCarthy, B. J., Davis, F. G., Preston-Martin, S. (2006) Descriptive epidemiology of vestibular schwannomas. *Neuro Oncol.*, 8:1 - 11.

[5] Preston, D. L, Ron, E., Yonehara, S., Kobuke, T., Fujii, H., Kishikawa, M. et al. (2002) Tumors of the nervous system and pituitary gland associated with atomic bomb radiation exposure. *J. Natl. Cancer Inst.*, 94: 1555 - 63.

[6] Yonehara, S., Brenner, A. V, Kishikawa, M., Inskip, P. D., Preston, D. L., Ron, E. et al. (2004) Clinical and epidemiologic characteristics of first primary tumors of the central nervous system and related organs among atomic bomb survivors in Hiroshima and Nagasaki, 1958 - 1995. *Cancer*, 101:1644 - 54.

[7] Mantao, C., Zuoxu, F., Xiujue, Z., Fei, C. and Liang, W. (2016). Risk Factors of Acoustic Neuroma: Systematic Review and Meta-Analysis. *Send to Yonsei Med. J.*, 57(3):776 - 83. doi: 10.3349/ ymj.2016.57.3.776.

[8] Martines, F., Giustino, V., Dispenza, F., Galletti, F., Iovane, A., Rizzo, S. and Messina, G. (2019). The Influence of Otovestibular System on Body Posture. *Advances in Audiology Research*, Nova Science Publishers, Inc. ISBN: 978-1-53615-260-9; in press.

[9] Giustino, V., Lo Russo, F., Rizzo, S., Salvago, P., Martines, F. (2019). Sudden sensorineural hearing loss. *Sensorineural Hearing Loss: Pathophysiology, Diagnosis and Treatment*, Nova Science Publishers, Inc. ISBN: 978-1-53615-048-3; in press.

[10] Thomas, E., Bianco, A., Messina, G., Mucia, M., Rizzo, S., Salvago, P., Sireci, F., Palma, A., Martines, F. (2017) The influence of sounds

in postural control. *Hearing Loss: Etiology, Management and Societal Implications,* pp. 1 - 11.

[11] Martines, F., Messina, G., Patti, A., Battaglia, G., Bellafiore, M., Messina, A., Rizzo, S., Salvago, P., Sireci, F., Traina, M., Iovane, A. (2015) Effects of tinnitus on postural control and stabilization: A pilot study. *Acta Medica Mediterranea*, 31: 907 - 912.

[12] Thomas, E., Martines, F., Bianco, A., Messina, G., Giustino, V., Zangla, D., Iovane, A., Palma, A. (2018) Decreased postural control in people with moderate hearing loss. *Medicine*, 97, 14, 1 DOI: 10.1097/MD.0000000000010244.

[13] Messina, G., Giustino, V., Dispenza, F., Galletti, F., Iovane, A., Rizzo, S. and Martines, F. (2019) Posturology: The Scientific Investigation of Postural Disorders. *Advances in Audiology Research*, Nova Science Publishers, Inc. ISBN: 978-1-53615-260-9; in press.

[14] Salvago, P., Rizzo, S., Bianco, A., Martines, F. (2017) Sudden sensorineural hearing loss: is there a relationship between routine haematological parameters and audiogram shapes? *International Journal of Audiology,* 56, 3, 148 - 153.

[15] Martines, F., Maira, E., Ferrara, S. (2011) Age-related hearing impairment (ARHI): A common sensory deficit in the elderly. *Acta Medica Mediterranea*, 27 (1), 47 - 52.

[16] Plescia, F., Cannizzaro, C., Brancato, A., Sireci, F., Salvago, P., Martines, F. (2016) Emerging pharmacological treatments of tinnitus. *Tinnitus: Epidemiology, Causes and Emerging Therapeutic Treatments*, pag. 43 - 64.

[17] Martines, F., Agrifoglio, M., Bentivegna, D., Mucia, M., Salvago, P., Sireci, F., Ballacchino, A. (2012) Treatment of tinnitus and dizziness associated vertebrobasilar insufficiency with a fixed combination of cinnarizine and dimenhydrinate. *Acta Medica Mediterranea*, 28 (3), 291 - 296.

[18] Rizzo, S., Sanfilippo, V., Terrana, P., Lauricella, L., Scaturro, D., Martines, F. and Letizia Mauro, G. (2019). Presbyastasis: from diagnosis to management *Sensorineural Hearing Loss:*

Pathophysiology, Diagnosis and Treatment, Nova Science Publishers, Inc. ISBN: 978-1-53615-048-3; in press.

[19] Cawthorne, T. (1944) The physiological basis of head exercises. *J. Chart. Soc. Physio. Ter.*, 30:106 - 7.

[20] Cooksey, F. S. (1946) Rehabilitation in vestibular injuries. *Proc. R. Soc. Physio. Med.*, 39: 273 - 8.

[21] Brandt, T. (1980) Physical Therapy for benign paroxysmal positional vertigo. *Arch. Otolaryngol.*, 106:484 - 485.

[22] Martines, F., Ballacchino, A., Sireci, F., Mucia, M., La Mattina, E., Rizzo, S., Salvago, P. (2016) Audiologic profile of OSAS and simple snoring patients: the effect of chronic nocturnal intermittent hypoxia on auditory function. *European Archives of Oto-Rhino-Laryngology,* 273, 6, 1419 - 1424.

[23] Ballacchino, A., Salvago, P., Cannizzaro, E., Costanzo, R., Di Marzo, M., Ferrara, S., La Mattina, E., Messina, G., Mucia, M., Mulè, A., Plescia, F., Sireci, F., Rizzo, S., Martines, F. (2015) Association between sleep-disordered breathing and hearing disorders: Clinical observation in Sicilian patients, *Acta Medica Mediterranea*, 31 (3), pp. 607 - 614.

[24] Dispenza, F., De Stefano, A., Costantino, C., Rando, D., Giglione, M., Stagno, R., Bennici, E. (2015) Canal switch and re-entry phenomenon in benign paroxysmal positional vertigo: difference between immediate and delayed occurrence. *Acta Otorhinolaryngol. Ital.*, 35: 116 - 120.

About the Editors

Francesco Dispenza MD, PhD
Otorhinolaryngology Department,
Policlinico University Hospital Palermo, Italy
Francesco.dispenza@gmail.com

Francesco Martines MD, PhD
BioNeC Department
University of Palermo, Italy
Francesco.martines@unipa.it

INDEX

L

M

N

O

P

R

S

T

U

V